RecordCovid19

RecordCovid19

Historicizing Experiences of the Pandemic

Edited by
Kristopher Lovell

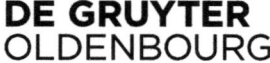
DE GRUYTER
OLDENBOURG

ISBN 978-3-11-073539-0
e-ISBN (PDF) 978-3-11-073100-2
e-ISBN (EPUB) 978-3-11-073111-8

Library of Congress Control Number: 2023937905

Bibliographic information published by the Deutsche Nationalbibliothek
The Deutsche Nationalbibliothek lists this publication in the Deutsche Nationalbibliografie;
detailed bibliographic data are available on the internet at http://dnb.dnb.de.

© 2023 Walter de Gruyter GmbH, Berlin/Boston
Cover image: Gettyimages/Feverpitched
Typesetting: Integra Software Services Pvt. Ltd.
Printing and binding: CPI books GmbH, Leck

www.degruyter.com

Contents

Kristopher Lovell
Introduction: *#RecordCovid19*

The *#RecordCovid19* research project, launched in March 2020, was inspired by an awareness of the growing international health crisis and an individual existential crisis. As the pandemic escalated, so did an insecurity regarding my own limitations and ability to contribute positively to evolving events. The heroic role of the historian during a pandemic is somewhat limited. There were no emergencies that required my particular skill set. As an historian of the wartime press, I was unlikely to be called upon to measure newspaper content. But as the international crisis unfolded – from the virus first being detected in December 2019, to being declared an outbreak by the World Health Organisation in January 2020, and then a pandemic in March, as the virus became more and more serious, with the British Government advising against non-essential travel in mid-March, to announcing the lockdown on 23 March – I wanted to contribute something. And so *#RecordCovid19* was established on 26 March 2020, the same day that the lockdown measures legally came into effect in the United Kingdom.

The aim of the *#RecordCovid19* project was to collect anonymous accounts from a range of people about their experiences during the pandemic. It was intended to be a future resource for generations to come. It hoped to record how people felt about the social and political responses to the virus. People's reactions to new stories from all over the world would depict how they coped with the prospect and realities of isolation. *#RecordCovid19* invited contributors to submit accounts about any aspect of their experience that they felt comfortable discussing. Submissions could be short form or long. Accounts were submitted anonymously but were published with a brief description provided by respondents themselves, based on what they felt comfortable sharing: Age, Gender, Occupation, Location.[1]

The aims of the project were inspired by my own research as a media historian of wartime Britain (1939–1945) in two ways. Firstly, it was inspired by the pioneering work of Mass Observation. Mass Observation was a social research organisation set up in 1937 with the aim of recording people's experiences of life in Britain by collecting diaries, accounts and questionnaires produced by volunteers. Mass Observation, as it explained to its respondents in 1941, sought to:

---

1 For example: [*#RecordCovid19*-1] Croydon, Civil Servant, Female, 25, https://kristopherlovell. com/2020/04/12/record-covid-19-1-croydon-civil-servant-female-25/, accessed 13 April 2023.

https://doi.org/10.1515/9783110731002-001

salvage history, both literally from the tin dustbin outside your door, and metaphorically from the equally ignoble end which it would suffer if it were allowed to lie fallow in people's memories until such a time after war as it became fashionable to write it up.[2]

#RecordCovid19 thus sought to provide people with the opportunity to contribute their accounts, based on their own experiences as they happened, to a repository that would record and preserve them, providing a collection of primary sources for historians and sociologists.

Secondly, the project was inspired by the works of Angus Calder (and by extension Roland Barthes), insofar as it sought to help future researchers trace the development of Covid-19 mythologies through time.[3] In the aftermath of the Second World War, as Calder demonstrates, individual wartime experiences were subsumed by a broader national narrative: nationally, the Myth of the Blitz suggested that wartime Britain was united, 'all in it together', and stoic in the face of war. Yet individual accounts written at the time reveal that for many in Britain, the war was a time of fear, racism, and division. Witnessing first-hand the days before lockdown in Britain, it seemed clear that several myths about life in the pandemic were starting to emerge in much the same way as the Myth of the Blitz developed, and some of the Covid-19 myths were even directly connected to the Myth of the Blitz. Grand narratives started to overshadow some of the smaller narratives. People claimed that the lockdown would show how Britain was once again 'all in it together' and how Britain with its Blitz Spirit would remain stoic in the face of Covid-19. Yet in the weeks and days before lockdown, pictures were being circulated of empty shelves in supermarket, stripped bare as some people were hoarding toilet rolls and pasta for themselves, often collecting food and goods that they could not possibly need (and much of which was later consigned wholesale to waste), at the cost of many others in need. By collecting accounts of life during the pandemic as it happened, the aim of *#RecordCovid19* was not to judge, disprove or debunk myths, but, it is hoped, to help future historians trace the development of these myths over time as they emerge.

---

2 Mass Observation File Report 869: 'Salvaging History', 11 September 1941, 9, https://www.massob servation.amdigital.co.uk/Documents/Details/FileReport-869?login=true, accessed 15 March 2023.
3 Angus Calder, *Myth of the Blitz* (London: Pimlico, 2006).

Themes of the Collection

This volume developed out of the themes that emerged from the *#RecordCovid19* collection and comprises chapters cultivated from an interdisciplinary range of contributors. Contributors were invited to submit chapters that were inspired by, but not limited by, the subjects that emerged from the submissions to *#RecordCovid19*.

The first chapter in this volume, by me as editor of the present volume and creator of the *#RecordCovid19* archive, seeks to provide an overview of the accounts submitted to the *#RecordCovid19* project in order to provide a greater context for the remaining chapters. It discusses the demographics of respondents as well as explores some of the themes that emerged from the accounts, with a particular focus on how respondents reacted to the realisation that they were living through an historic moment in time and places this incredulity within a wider context. In so doing, it also highlights some of the challenges that historians still face in convincing individuals that their voices are important to history.

The rest of the edited volume is divided broadly into sections that reflect this contextualisation: experiences, rhetoric and narratives. The work builds from discussions of the practical implications of living through the pandemic, to the official and unofficial ways in which the health crisis was communicated before exploring the ways in which these stories shaped, and were shaped by, the pandemic.

The first section starts with Josephine Hoegaerts' examination of an often-overlooked aspect of historical experience: one's relationship with the soundscapes that make up the background of our quotidian existence. Through a detailed examination of accounts submitted to *#RecordCovid19*, Hoegaerts explores how people's relationship with sounds changed during the pandemic and explores how perceptions of sound and space are often culturally and historically framed. It also critically raises some key questions about how accurately sound (and the perception of sound) can be recorded and the exciting challenges these pose to historians of sounds.

Chapter Three analyses the impact of the pandemic on the various stages of pregnancy and early parenthood. Elizabeth Benjamin and Sarah Turner use socio-cultural and auto-ethnographic approaches to demonstrate that while the pandemic imposed great changes upon us all, those shifting their familial composition were particularly strongly affected. The chapter focuses on parental roles while recognising the disproportionate burden put on women both during and outside of the pandemic, and both within and outside of motherhood.

In the fourth chapter, Iro Filippaki and Alexandra Palli employ an interdisciplinary, psycho-historical perspective to examine, through an exploration of responses to questionnaires from Greek psychiatric patients, the varying emotional responses to the pandemic, and the ways in which this might affect people's response to other illnesses. It particularly focuses on the role emotions have in narratives of resilience, examining the role of empathy in the development of narratives of resilience.

The second section critically examines the rhetoric surrounding Covid-19 in Britain's responses to the pandemic. Christopher Smith explores, in the fifth chapter, the political use of references to Britain's experience of the Second World War in the UK government's narratives aimed at the population. The chapter builds on a discussion of the Myth of the Blitz, and demonstrates a thematic paradox, namely: that while the use of war myth narrative was strong in government messaging, the resonance was surprisingly low among the participants in the *#RecordCovid19* project.

Chapter Six, by Franziska E. Kohlt, engages in a critical examination of how the British political responses framed the pandemic around religious rhetoric and how the religious framing of the pandemic often emerged from the rhetoric of war. Kohlt highlights how whilst these rhetorical references might have chimed with the British public in the short-term, they often had a detrimental and dangerous impact long term. In so doing, this chapter provides some insights into how future pandemics and health-crises should be communicated.

The final section explores the construction of narratives. In Chapter Seven, Darren Reid discusses how in extraordinary times ordinary people become storytellers as well as active consumers of stories. Storytelling during the pandemic became a form of catharsis: this catharsis was often characterised and influenced by wider narratives in popular media. The chapter demonstrates how escapism was often essential for many individuals to ground their historical experience of the pandemic.

In the final chapter, Arddun Arwyn offers an examination of the construction of narratives in times of crisis and the ways in which individual stories are rarely truly individual. Shared narratives often help individuals and communities make sense of the moments they live through but, as Arwyn demonstrates, researchers interested in using primary accounts taken during such times should critically be aware of the fact that these narratives tell us more about the truth of how people felt in the moment but do not necessarily accurately relate the facts of an event. This chapter historically problematises the *#RecordCovid19* archive through its discussion of narrative tropes that emerged from German expellees in the post-war era and provides a clear insight into how researchers should use these accounts.

These chapters, along with the accounts submitted to the project, reveal the wide range of experiences that people faced during the pandemic. They also show the extent to which a universal event is experienced differently by everyone involved.

From the conception of the project, the *#RecordCovid19* archive was always intended to be an open and publicly available archive. An archive that allowed people to share experiences, by submitting accounts themselves or by reading through the accounts of others. The project wanted to avoid capturing people's memories only to lock them away in private archives out of the reach of the public – or worse, charge participants for the right to read the research derived from their contributions. De Gruyter, and Rabea Rittgerodt, have helped make that ambition a reality by allowing us to put together this edited collection that hopes to historicize the pandemic.[4]

#RecordCovid19 is a small project. It was intended only to record a small drop in an ocean of experiences related to Covid-19. It has, however, been immensely gratifying that some respondents found a few moments of comfort in contributing their words to *#RecordCovid19*. As one contributor wrote, 'Writing here kind of helps me to clear my thoughts and at least give me some motivation about the way life is these days';[5] another commented that 'I hope this project gets published in some way. I have found relief in reading these entries over the course of the lockdown – thank you for providing that'.[6]

#RecordCovid19 is not intended to be *the* archive of Covid-19 experience – the project is intended record a moment of living history and collective memory. I hope that it provides an insight into the myriad of experiences that made up the pandemic and one that can be used in conjunction with other existing and future collections.

---

4 The accounts submitted to the *#RecordCovid19* project can be read for free here: https://kristo pherlovell.com/category/recordcovid19-project/.

5 [*#RecordCovid19*-112] Turkey, Student, Female, 20, https://kristopherlovell.com/2021/01/31/record covid19-112-turkey-student-female-20/, accessed 13 April 2023.

6 [*#RecordCovid19*-68] London, Female, Civil Servant, 25–30, https://kristopherlovell.com/2020/06/25/recordcovid19-68-london-female-civil-servant-25-30/, accessed 13 April 2023.

Kristopher Lovell

Chapter One
History Happens To Other People?
Memory, Myth and History in
#RecordCovid19

Introduction

At once exciting and exhilarating, traumatic and terrifying, history can feel very distant, or it can feel a little too close. For many, history is not something they feel they have to worry about. But as American author Philip Roth notes, 'History claims everybody, whether they know it or not and whether they like it or not.'[1] As Covid-19 spread throughout the world, many who had felt that history normally passed them by increasingly felt a part of it. In our ever-mediatised world, people simultaneously witnessed and experienced historic events as they unfolded.

This chapter provides an overview of the *#RecordCovid19* project, drawing upon the themes and issues presented by individual contributors and detailing what the project tells us about the gamut of experiences of respondents living through history within a wider context of cultural trauma and collective memory. The first section discusses Covid-19 as a moment of historic memory and cultural trauma and the role of the modern media in shaping, framing and sharing experiences. The second section provides a demographic overview of the respondents who submitted accounts to *#RecordCovid19*. Section three explores some of the dominant themes that emerge from the accounts. Finally, this chapter highlights some of the limitations of the project before considering some of the lessons of *#RecordCovid19*.

This chapter explores how – through the case study of responses collected through the *#RecordCovid19* project – people reacted to the realisation that they were experiencing a distinct moment in history. As such, it offers its own snapshot of time, assessing two years of responses to a global pandemic as it happened, as it relates to our collective framing of crisis.

---

[1] Philip Roth, 'The Story Behind "The Plot Against America,"' *The New York Times*, 19 September 2004, 10–12, https://www.nytimes.com/2004/09/19/books/review/the-story-behind-the-plot-against-america.html?smid=url-share, accessed 13 April 2023.

https://doi.org/10.1515/9783110731002-002

Memory, Cultural Trauma and Covid-19

Whilst memory is fundamental to how we perceive ourselves,[2] it is also essential for creating societal bonds.[3] Memory is not static, however. As Schacter and Welker note, memory is 'a dynamic, constructive process that reflects the goals and biases of individuals and groups, rather than a static or literal reproduction of past experiences.[4]

The field of memory studies has noted the development of 'memory booms' that have coincided with developments in communication technology, culminating recently in the 'connective turn' which includes, according to Hoskins:

> the enveloping of the everyday in real-time or near-instantaneous communications, including 'messaging', be these peer-to-peer, one-to-many, or more complex and diffused connections within and between groups, 'crowds', or networks, and facilitated through mobile media and social networking technologies and other internet-based services.[5]

The ways in which the media frames events shapes both individual and collective memory thereof. In fact, historically the media has often shaped the narratives that exist in collective memory.

The framing of events by the media includes what is referred to in cognitive psychology as 'flashbulb memories.'[6] This refers to a phenomenon with which we are now intimately familiar: the hearing or seeing of an event through the media. As Andrew Hoskins notes, 'the potential influence of the mass media in shaping memory is related to the idea of a mass audience in forging a collective (often simultaneous) reception of an event.'[7] This also establishes cultural trauma – when the experience of a tragic or momentous event 'leaves indelible marks upon their group consciousness, marking their memories forever and changing their future identity in fundamental and irrevocable ways.'[8]

---

2 Yadin Dudai and Micha Edelson, 'Personal Memory: Is It Personal, Is It Memory?' *Memory Studies*, 9:3 (2016), 275. https://doi.org/10.1177/1750698016645234.

3 Daniel L. Schacter and Michael Welker, 'Memory and Connection: Remembering the Past and Imagining the Future in Individuals, Groups, and Cultures,' *Memory Studies*, 9:3 (July 2016): 241–244. https://doi.org/10.1177/1750698016645229.

4 Daniel Schachter and Michael Welker, 'Memory And Connection: Remembering The Past And Imagining The Future In Individuals, Groups, And Cultures,' *Memory Studies* 9:3 (2016), 241.

5 Andrew Hoskins 'Media, Memory, Metaphor: Remembering and the Connective Turn', *Parallax* 17:4, (2011), 20. https://doi.org/10.1080/13534645.2011.605573.

6 Andrew Hoskins, 'The Restless Past: An Introduction To Digital Memory And Media,' in *Digital Media Studies*, ed. by Andrew Hoskins (NY: Taylor and Francis, 2018), 17.

7 Hoskins, 'The Restless Past,' 17.

8 Jeffrey C. Alexander, 'Toward a Theory of Cultural Trauma,' in. *Cultural Trauma and Collective Identity*, eds. Jeffrey C Alexander et al. (University of California Press, 2004), 1, https://ebookcentral.proquest.com/lib/coventry/detail.action?docID=837285, accessed 13 April 2023.

The combination of the connective turn and a pandemic has led to a moment of cultural trauma hitherto unseen. The incessant nature of the internet means that experiences and memories are constantly being recorded, erased and changed. As Geoffrey Cubitt notes:

> From materials and messages that are transmitted within society, specific representations and larger understandings of a collective past are continuously woven. Events, experiences and personalities that have left an impact in people's thinking get incorporated into narratives or organised accounts of society's or the nation's past.[9]

However, when the broader narratives are developed they often overshadow – and sometimes erase – the individual experiences. The rise of the Global Village, as McLuhan put it, also allows memories to be shared in real time across the world;[10] it also allows (or even forces) societies to share trauma transnationally. This is, of course, not restricted to the experience of Covid-19. Cultural trauma has been shared during acts of terror and violence – notably it was seen in the wake of the 2015 attacks on Paris, as global citizens of social media claimed '#JeSuisCharlie' or overlaid the French flag over their usual profile picture.[11]

Collective memories of historical events are often used by the media and government to frame current events. This was true during the Covid-19 pandemic in Britain, which saw the collective memory of the Second World War regularly invoked, in particular the notion of the Blitz Spirit: Britain's mythic resilience in the face of war. As early as March 2020, Britain's Health Secretary Matt Hancock openly invoked the memory of the Blitz:

> Our generation has never been tested like this. Our grandparents were, during the Second World War, when our cities were bombed during the Blitz. Despite the pounding every night, the rationing, the loss of life, they pulled together in one gigantic national effort.[12]

A month later, the Queen similarly framed her broadcast to the nation with a rhetoric of war as she compared the imposition of social distancing to wartime evacuation, before promising the British public that, just like after the war, 'We'll

---

9 Geoffrey Cubitt, *History and Memory* (Manchester: MUP, 2007), 199.

10 See for example: Marshall McLuhan, *The Gutenberg Galaxy: The Making of Typographic Man* (Toronto: University of Toronto Press, 1962).

11 For a more detailed discussion of this case, see Johnny Alam's chapter in Laura Macaluso (2019): Johnny Alam, 'Transnational Social Media Monuments, Counter-Monuments, and Future of the Nation-State,' in *Monument Culture: International Perspectives on the Future of Monuments in a Changing World,* ed. by Laura Macaluso (London: Rowman & Littlefield, 2019), 191–204.

12 'News Story: Health Secretary Matt Hancock's Sunday Telegraph Op-Ed', 15 March 2020, https://www.gov.uk/government/news/health-secretary-matt-hancocks-sunday-telegraph-op-ed, accessed 13 April 2023.

Meet Again'.[13] These were not isolated cases of the memory of the war being manipulated to this effect. British newspapers, the *Daily Telegraph* in particular,[14] regularly evoked the spirit of the Blitz during the pandemic.[15] This narrative helped frame the experience but as will be explored later in this chapter, it has overshadowed the gamut of experiences respondents have felt since 2020.

#RecordCovid19 Respondents

As Emil Durkheim notes, 'when society is going through events that sadden, distress, or anger it, it pushes its members to give witness to their sadness, distress, or anger through expressive actions.'[16] People living through historic moments often feel compelled to record for posterity their experiences. The connective turn also allows people to use social media to share their experiences in real time. *#RecordCovid19* was one project that sought to collect experiences and memories of the pandemic and the feeling of living through an historic moment.

As of May 2022, *#RecordCovid19* has received 119 accounts. The majority of the accounts (71; 60%) were submitted by respondents who identified themselves as female, whereas 27 accounts (23%) were submitted by respondents who identified as male. 15 respondents chose not to disclose their gender, 4 identified as non-binary, 1 as genderfluid and 1 as genderqueer. Of course, one needs to be mindful that these figures include respondents with multiple submissions, so it is not necessarily the case that 71 women submitted accounts, but rather that 71 accounts were submitted by women. Still, it is clear that women were much more likely to submit accounts to *#RecordCovid19* than men. This gender disparity is not restricted to this project. In fact, several similar projects appear to have corresponding divisions in gender. The Collecting Covid Questionnaire 2020, run by *Amgueddfa Cymru,* received responses from 1019 respondents, 79% of which were from female respondents.[17] The Young

---

13 Caroline Davies, '"We Will Meet Again": Queen Urges Britons To Stay Strong,' *The Guardian*, 5 April 2020, https://www.theguardian.com/world/2020/apr/05/queen-urges-britons-stay-strong-coronavirus-covid-lockdown, accessed 14 April 2023.

14 Anon., 'Blitz Spirit is Back: Meet The Covid-19 Heroes,' *Daily Telegraph*, 28 March 2020, 5.

15 Deliberate referencing of the Second World War is covered in more detail in Christopher Smith's chapter in this collection.

16 Emile Durkheim, *The Elementary Forms of Religious Life* (London: The Free Press, 1995), 415. Translated Karen E. Fields.

17 Arad Research, *Collecting Covid Questionnaire 2020: Analysis of Responses: Final Report* (August 2021), 26,https://museum.wales/media/53025/Collecting-Covid-2020_English_Final.pdf, accessed 13 April 2023.

Foundation's *Covid and You* project received approximately 600 respondents, 75% of which were submitted by female respondents. In terms of age distribution, the average age of a *#RecordCovid19* respondent was 27 years, with the youngest account submitted by a 17-year-old and the oldest by a 75-year-old. Broken down by gender, the average age of a female respondent was 29 years and 24 years old for male respondents. The majority of accounts were submitted by women in their twenties with 96 of the accounts from women aged 30 or under.

Geographically, the majority of the entries were submitted by people living in the UK. At the time of writing, 76 of the accounts came from the UK with the majority (55) coming from England, followed by Wales (20), and only a single account from Northern Ireland. 12 accounts were submitted from Turkey (where it appears to have been set as an assignment by a teacher). 7 came from the US. 4 were submitted from 'abroad' and the rest were submitted from France, Australia, Germany, Iceland, Canada, Philippines and Finland.

In terms of occupation, 47 of the respondents were from various types of students studying a range of subjects, from history to medicine. 10 were from teachers across the country. There were a small number of civil servants, writers, engineers and diplomats. It is worth noting that this is a very self-selecting sample by nature. It seems that the average *#RecordCovid19* participant was educated, liberal, and young. This reveals a slight irony in the ambitions of the project (see introduction). In the attempt to emulate the work of Mass Observation, *#RecordCovid19* also emulated one of Mass Observation's shortfalls – its focus on educated, liberal and young diarists. But all projects of this sort are self-selecting – they depend on someone being historically minded and aware of the importance of the moment they are recording. It also relies on someone wanting to share their stories to be preserved for the future, which again tends to be a sign that someone has an interest in history.

Themes from *#RecordCovid19*

The experience of life under lockdown elicited a variety of responses from people. Accounts submitted to the project varied greatly in length, with some being little more than a few sentences and others being pages long. In total over 55,000 words were submitted to the project. This allowed respondents to submit accounts in a form that they felt best expressed their experiences. Respondents discussed a wide range of issues in their accounts and each account was idiosyncratic, even when they discussed similar aspects or covered similar themes. This section will introduce a few of the major themes that emerged from the accounts before focusing specifically on how respondents felt about living through history.

Many accounts understandably talked about the impact that lockdown had on their lives, displaying a gamut of reactions to confinement and isolation. Some respondents were deeply distressed by the prospect of lockdown alone. A female engineer from Wales on 12 April 2020 struggled with the prospect of isolation. 'I don't want to be alone. I don't want to be stuck in the top floor of a building.'[18] The decision where to spend lockdown was also a source of contention and frustration. 'It's been hard being split up from loved ones', one female respondent from Coventry wrote, 'and even worse when your loved one made the decision to go home to be with their family which include someone who needs to shield.'[19]

The submissions reveal that the experience of lockdown life varied greatly. For some, the pandemic provided them with the opportunity to learn new skills and hone their talents. One young respondent from Chester used the lockdown to start exercising and learning a language: 'I really want to use this opportunity', he wrote, 'to better myself as much as we can in these situations.'[20] Another, a diplomat working abroad claimed that despite working incessantly, lockdown for her was 'like a holiday' because 'all boundaries between work and time off have been dissolved even further.'[21] A female admin worker from Walsall felt that isolation 'brought out a great sense of fun and creativity in others.'[22] Some felt conflicted, partly because their circumstances allowed them to enjoy themselves. As one respondent, a freelancer from Wales, wrote:

> I'm now vacillating between happiness and guilt: I am loving the freedom of doing little, doing it well, gardening, cooking, enjoying the sun, the wind, the growth; but feeling guilty that I am lucky to have a great place to be, space, garden, some savings and another person to isolate both with and from.[23]

---

18 [*#RecordCovid19*–5] Wales, Engineer, Female, 30, https://kristopherlovell.com/2020/04/13/re cord-covid-19-5-wales-engineer-female-30/, accessed 13 April 2023.

19 [*#RecordCovid19*–74] Coventry, Admin, Female, 22, https://kristopherlovell.com/2020/07/07/re cordcovid19-73-coventry-admin-female-22/, accessed 13 April 2023.

20 [*#RecordCovid19*–11] Chester, Student, Male, 21, https://kristopherlovell.com/2020/04/17/record-covid-19-11-chester-student-male-21/, accessed 13 April 2023.

21 [*#RecordCovid19*–21] Abroad, Diplomat, Female, 30–35, https://kristopherlovell.com/2020/04/24/record-covid19-21-abroad-diplomat-female-30-35/, accessed 13 April 2023.

22 [*#RecordCovid19*–30] Walsall, Admin, F, 45, https://kristopherlovell.com/2020/04/27/record-covid19-30-walsall-admin-f-45/, accessed 13 April 2023.

23 [*#RecordCovid19*–6] West Wales, Freelance Teacher, Trainer, Project Manager, Female. 61, https://kristopherlovell.com/2020/04/14/record-covid-19-6-west-wales-freelance-teacher-trainer-project-manager-female-61/, accessed 13 April 2023.

However, much like how the impact of the pandemic placed some lives more at risk than others depending on class, gender and age, the lockdown affected some social lives more than others too. Those with more secure incomes or whose jobs were included in the furlough schemes could see lockdown was an opportunity.

Naturally, these positive attitudes were not universal, and they greatly depended on the circumstances of the individual. Many struggled with the restrictions placed upon their social lives. Others found the experience of the lockdown exhausting and destructive. A trainee English teacher felt that time had been compressed, and 'With little to differentiate between weekday and weekend, I often found myself partaking in drinking games . . .'[24] Poignantly, a postgraduate student struggling with the pandemic and their workload despaired:

> I am breaking.
> No.
> Broken.[25]

The discrepancy between experiences was even noted by some of the respondents. 'I'm sick of the relentless optimists who keep trying to tout this whole lockdown period as some fecund field of personal growth', a female writer from Wales reported. 'It's not. We can't all spend our time meditating and making sourdough bread . . .'[26] The differences in lockdown experiences could also affect personal relationships, especially if the lived experience differed greatly within households. An admin worker from Coventry envied her partner's time on furlough. 'My furloughed friends and families have been taking the time to learn, better themselves, protest and have days sunbathing in the park, whilst I hunch over my laptop in the corner of a darkened room.'[27] Some who enjoyed lockdown even felt guilty because they were in a privileged position to be able to enjoy, either because of where they lived (countryside versus city), the type of work they did or simply because they

---

24 [*#RecordCovid19*–72] Essex, Trainee English Teacher, Male, 23, https://kristopherlovell.com/2020/07/01/recordcovid19-72-essex-trainee-english-teacher-male-23/, accessed 13 April 2023.
25 [*#RecordCovid19*–109] Brighton, Postgrad Student, Male, https://kristopherlovell.com/2021/01/14/recordcovid19-109-brighton-postgrad-student-male/, accessed 13 April 2023.
26 [*#RecordCovid19*–50] Wales, Writer, Female, 28, https://kristopherlovell.com/2020/05/10/recordcovid19-50-wales-writer-female-28/, accessed 13 April 2023.
27 [*#RecordCovid19*–69] Coventry, Admin Worker, Female, 22, https://kristopherlovell.com/2020/06/28/recordcovid19-69-coventry-admin-worker-female-22/, accessed 13 April 2023.

had lots of entertainment available to them at home.[28] Some were able to relativise their situation, recognising that whilst they were struggling, they were 'lucky to be privileged enough to avoid the horrors of the real world.'[29]

History Happens to Other People?

One theme that emerged early on in the project surrounded the experience of respondents as they realised they were living through a moment of history. As early as 24 March 2020, the day after Boris Johnson's speech announcing the lockdown, a civil servant from Croydon noted that she felt that they were living through 'a bad dream, a history book, or some apocalyptic film.'[30] Naturally, students of history were particularly susceptible to this feeling. One such respondent stated that they 'study history for a reason. I never thought I'd be living through a major event in it.'[31] This feeling was not an isolated one. Another female history student from Lincoln wrote: 'It feels very strange to know that I am living through something that will be remembered in history and eventually taught to students. I never really thought I would live through anything significant like this.'[32] Even respondents who wanted to be eyewitnesses to history seemed to regret the type of history they found themselves experiencing. After learning about major events like the March on Washington for Jobs and Freedom, one respondent admitted to wishing to be a participant of history, but not this type of history: 'I never envisaged that my notable historical experience to be a mass pandemic.'[33]

The degree of disbelief about living through an important moment varied. Occasionally respondents expressed disbelief that not only were they living through *a* major historical event but they were living through *multiple* events simultaneously, specifically living through the pandemic and the BlackLivesMatter protests. As one

---

28 [*#RecordCovid19*–98] West Wales, freelance teacher, trainer, project manager, Female, now 62, https://kristopherlovell.com/2020/10/20/recordcovid19-98-west-wales-freelance-teacher-trainer-project-manager-female-now-62/, accessed 13 April 2023.
29 [*#RecordCovid19*–118] Birmingham, Male, 21, https://kristopherlovell.com/2021/09/02/recordcovid19-118-birmingham-male-21/, accessed 13 April 2023.
30 [*#RecordCovid19*–1] Croydon, Civil Servant, Female, 25, https://kristopherlovell.com/2020/04/12/record-covid-19-1-croydon-civil-servant-female-25/, accessed 13 April 2023.
31 [*#RecordCovid19*–10] Swindon, Student, Female, 22, https://kristopherlovell.com/2020/04/17/record-covid19-10-swindon-student-female-22/, accessed 13 April 2023.
32 [*#RecordCovid19*–12] Lincolnshire, History Student, Female, 20, https://kristopherlovell.com/2020/04/17/record-covid-19-12-lincolnshire-history-student-female-20/, accessed 13 April 2023.
33 [*#RecordCovid19*–13] Lincolnshire, Student, Female, 21, https://kristopherlovell.com/2020/04/18/record-covid-19-13-lincolnshire-student-female-21/, accessed 13 April 2023.

female student from Ontario noted: 'I don't know why. I know that doesn't really make sense, and that major events can obviously happen concurrently, but reading or learning about this in regards to history is so different than actually living it.'[34]

This perception was not just restricted to history students; there was a broader realisation that people were living through history. It seems that this feeling provided some with comfort and clarity. Thinking of the pandemic as a future historical event helped some to deal with its challenges. A hairstylist from the US noted: 'I know I'm living through a chapter in a history book. It's strange, but I can almost disconnect myself from this reality when I think of it like that.' The comfort for this respondent was that historical events felt less threatening when they were viewed as historical:

> 'This isn't going to be real for someone. This will be a paragraph in a book, a question on a test that someone is anxious about. This will be 20 different movies, all with the same plot that kids roll their eyes at, dozens of books about finding love in quarantine. This won't be real someday.'
> And for just a few moments, it isn't real.
> God, I wish this wasn't real.[35]

This comfort was not restricted to just one or two isolated voices, although the reasons for their comfort varied. History, to one respondent at least, was full of events that they perceived as far more threatening than Covid-19. Perhaps drawing on the fact the 1918 Influenza Pandemic (commonly referred to as the Spanish Flu) has been largely forgotten in popular memory, a couple of respondents predicted that a similar reaction would happen to Covid-19. A male office worker from Sweden claimed:

> I compartmentalize covid, i take it in strides, i'm doing alright. Looking through the history books covid is hardly worth a foot note. We've seen so much worse, things that we can't even pretend to understand the darkness of. But i hope for the sake of all those that don't feel fine, that covid will soon be over [sic].[36]

A similar sentiment was echoed by another who hoped that the feeling of solidary that existed at the start of the pandemic would last long after it was over, however they feared that most would strive to forget about it and there would be no lessons learnt from the experience. A financial worker from Derry feared:

---

34 [*#RecordCovid19*–66] Ontario Canada, Student, Female, 21, https://kristopherlovell.com/2020/06/16/recordcovid19-66-ontario-canada-student-female-21/, accessed 13 April 2023.
35 [*#RecordCovid19*–20] USA, Hairstylist, Female, 21, https://kristopherlovell.com/2020/04/24/record-covid19-20-usa-hairstylist-female-21/, accessed 13 April 2023.
36 [*#RecordCovid19*–101] Sweden, Office Worker, Male 28, https://kristopherlovell.com/2020/11/02/recordcovid19-101-sweden-office-worker-male-28/, accessed 13 April 2023.

we'll cover up the cracks that Covid has exposed instead of taking positive steps to fix them. I realise that the pandemic is but a fleeting moment in history and that nothing lasts forever, I also realise people who it has effected will last far beyond Covid's brief span.[37]

The experience of the pandemic would be lost in the noise of history just as many other big moments of history have been forgotten or relegated to the epilogues of many books.

The act of remembering the event and how it could be presented in the future was an issue that some *#RecordCovid19* accounts considered. In particular, some wondered how the experience of the pandemic might be commemorated in museums, and what lessons future generations might make of it. Of course, these accounts are conjecture – speculations about which ephemeral objects, such as official government letters or newspapers, would be chosen for historical prosperity in order to show their children one day or what might be 'shoved into a glass display cabinet and labelled 'Covid-19 pandemic, 2020'[38] – but the process of thinking about tomorrow's history seems to have provided a moment of respite from the predicament of the present. An unemployed female respondent from the UK claimed:

I like thinking about the future, because it's a distraction from the monotony of the present. I hate thinking about the future, because it's such an uncertain thing, and it will either be brilliant or terrible or both.[39]

Another account, from a history student, speculated that the impact of the pandemic would affect many generations to come and will be a subject of much historical discussion in the future: 'there are many people who doubt the importance of History of a subject [sic], I hope this epidemic allows you to learn, to further your knowledge, that we cannot return to "normality", and finally, History does repeat itself.'[40] The experience of living through an event reassured them of the value of history.

The experience of the pandemic also helped some to understand and appreciate societies in the past a little more. One student of history explained in their account that they had never understood or appreciated 'the rather deep relationship

---

37 [*#RecordCovid19*–103] Derry, Financial Services Analyst, 24 https://kristopherlovell.com/2020/11/03/recordcovid19-102-derry-financial-services-analyst-24/, accessed 13 April 2023.
38 [*#RecordCovid19*–10] Swindon, Student, Female, 22 https://kristopherlovell.com/2020/04/17/record-covid19-10-swindon-student-female-22/, accessed 13 April 2023; [*#RecordCovid19*–75] UK, Unemployed (the current national occupation), Female, 28, https://kristopherlovell.com/2020/07/19/record covid19-74-uk-unemployed-the-current-national-occupation-female-28/, accessed 13 April 2023.
39 [*#RecordCovid19*–75] UK, Unemployed (the current national occupation), Female, 28, https://kristopherlovell.com/2020/07/19/recordcovid19-74-uk-unemployed-the-current-national-occupa tion-female-28/, accessed 13 April 2023.
40 [*#RecordCovid19*–26] Newport South Wales, MA student, Female, 22, https://kristopherlovell.com/2020/04/25/record-covid19-26-newport-south-wales-ma-student-female-22/.

between a Prime Minister and the state of public attitude during war, or times of great strain', but during the pandemic they began to appreciate it more as they sought comfort from seeing Prime Minister Boris Johnson and Dominic Raab during their press conferences.[41]

Interestingly these feelings are not restricted to *#RecordCovid19* and can be seen in other accounts from comparable projects. For example, Swansea University's *CoronaDiary Project* also showcases the range of responses from people to realising that history was something they were living through.[42] This reaction started quite early on in the British experience of the pandemic. One account from young diarist, Remi, explains that they were participating in the project because they were 'experiencing the effects of the global pandemic which will go down in history and no doubt be referred to in films, books, tv series and all sorts.' Interestingly, it was the media depiction of past historical events that helped Remi realise the historical gravity of the situation ('You could say that Spanish Flu episode of Downton Abbey inspired me').[43] The following month, a respondent named Owen recorded a 'sense of being at a crossroads in history' that might potentially bring changes to society comparable to those that followed the two World Wars.[44]

Again this was not isolated to just one diarist in the project but there are several accounts that discuss the surprise about living through historic moments. Diarist Diane wrote directly to her readers in the future explaining how she felt about the experience: 'So those of you reading this in the future and looking on this pandemic as history I can say I haven't felt as if I have been part of a historical event'.[45] Instead for her, she was simply trying to get through it. Other diarists struggled with perceiving the pandemic as historical because of the uncertainty it brought. Brooke, in March 2020, expressed fear about what the future will be after living through 'one of those seminal moments in history'.[46]

---

41 [*#RecordCovid19*–43] Student, Female, 20, https://kristopherlovell.com/2020/05/01/record-covid19-43-student-female-20/, accessed 13 April 2023.

42 Michael Ward, 'CoronaDiaries: Documenting The Everyday Lived Experiences Of A Global Pandemic,' https://collections.swansea.ac.uk/s/coronadiaries/page/home, accessed 13 April 2023.

43 Remi, Female, aged 18–24, University Student, Indian, Single, living with family during lockdown, 18 March 2020, https://collections.swansea.ac.uk/s/coronadiaries/page/Remi#?c=0&m=0&s=0&cv=0, accessed 13 April 2023.

44 Owen, Male, aged 45–54, 25 April 2020, https://collections.swansea.ac.uk/s/coronadiaries/page/Owen#?c=0&m=0&s=0&cv=0, accessed 13 April 2023.

45 Diane, Female, aged 55–64, Retired University Administrator, Southeast England, 30 March 2021, https://collections.swansea.ac.uk/s/coronadiaries/page/Diane#?c=0&m=0&s=0&cv=0, accessed 13 April 2023.

46 Brooke, Female, aged 25–34, PHD Student 17 March 2020, https://collections.swansea.ac.uk/s/coronadiaries/page/Brooke, accessed 13 April 2023.

The disbelief (and sudden realisation) that we are living through a historic moment is not new either. There are countless examples throughout history of witnesses expressing disbelief at being part of (or at least witnessing) major historical events. Stefan Zweig, for example, an Austrian novelist and journalist who recorded the rise of Nazi Germany in his autobiography, considered it 'an iron law of history that those who will be caught up in the great movements determining the course of their own times always fail to recognise them in their early stages.'[47]

Historians and journalists have previously attempted to engage with the wide range of feelings about living through moments of history (and the challenge of being an historian living through it). In the aftermath of the September 11 attacks, *New York Times'* Sam Roberts interviewed Kenneth T. Jackson, president of the Historical Society, about the moment when living through an experience becomes history and when it becomes acceptable for an historian to intervene and record it. Jackson admits that he wished he had collected some ephemeral artefacts at the time because '. . . historians have a duty to preserve', but in the case of September 11 as 'this was a crime scene, historians, in a certain sense, were pushed out.'[48] Journalist Masha Gessen, writing for the *New Yorker*, also pondered about the historical condition. In her discussion about the use of the phrase 'concentration camps' to describe US detention camps in 2019, Green warned of the dangers of history becoming distorted:

> We learn to think of history as something that has already happened, to other people. Our own moment, filled as it is with minutiae destined to be forgotten, always looks smaller in comparison. As for history, the greater the event, the more mythologized it becomes. Despite our best intentions, the myth becomes a caricature of sorts.[49]

Ameila Tait, journalist for The *New Statesman*, reflected on her experience witnessing an anti-Brexit protest.

> We are all always living through history. Yet there are times in our lives when we are acutely aware that we are witnessing something significant – or in my case, when I feel as though I'm living in the "Causes" chapter of a teenager's GCSE history book, even if I don't yet know what is going to be caused.[50]

---

47 Stefan Zweig, *The World Of Yesterday*, (London: Puskin Press, 2009) Kindle Edition, 310.

48 Sam Roberts, 'When History Isn't Something That Happens to Other People,' *New York Times*, 24 April 2002, 15, https://www.nytimes.com/2002/04/24/arts/when-history-isn-t-something-that-happens-to-other-people.html, accessed 13 April 2023.

49 Masha Gessen, 'The Unimaginable Reality of American Concentration Camps,' *New Yorker*, 21 June 2019,https://www.newyorker.com/news/our-columnists/the-unimaginable-reality-of-american-concentration-camps, accessed 13 April 2023.

50 Amelia Tait, 'We Think Of History As Something That Happened To Other People, But We're Living Through It Every Day,' *The New Statesman*, 13 June 2012, https://www.newstatesman.com/

What is striking about all of these examples is that the feeling remains pervasive: those who lived through historic moments seemingly forget they lived through history as soon as a greater moment in history arises. Many of the *#RecordCovid19* accounts referenced above, in which participants expressed surprise at living through history, were from respondents who lived in Britain during the Brexit referendum and debate but this has seemingly been overshadowed by the pandemic.

As this project was partly inspired by Mass Observation's attempts to record the Second World War, it is perhaps pertinent to end with an example from the period which demonstrates the persistence of this feeling (and perhaps its relationship with the media). On 14 April 1939, the *Yorkshire Evening Post*, a British provincial newspaper, discussed the prospect of a new world war breaking out. The editors of the paper were just as uncertain about the future as anyone else was and were just as uncertain about the prospect of finding themselves living through history:

> What we are painfully aware of is the fact that history (on the present example) is a good deal more agreeable to read about than to live through. In history (if it is sufficiently remote) we can at any time learn the sequel – and yet how ironical if we go on to say that "those were the days!". These are the days enough for anybody, and there will be fine chapters written about them eventually; we may even be envied for the times we lived through and for the colour and excitement and the challenge there was in our lives. But it isn't an attitude of mind that is very easy to adopt just now; we would, in short, prefer to do without some of the chapters that will absorb the eventual student, and know the end of the story.[51]

The staff at the *Yorkshire Evening Post* would of course find themselves living through many chapters of history during the Second World War. And, very ironically indeed, the age they found themselves living through has been viewed nostalgically in modern Britain.

Conclusion

What conclusions can be drawn from the *#RecordCovid19* archive? Firstly, the archive clearly shows that the experience of living through various aspects of the pandemic differed greatly between people, households and communities. It might be assumed that living through the pandemic's lockdowns and isolation was a

---

politics/uk-politics/2012/06/we-think-history-something-happened-other-people-we-re-living-through-it-every, accessed 13 April 2023.
51 Leader, 'On Knowing the End,' *Yorkshire Evening Post*, 14 April 1939, 10.

universal experience – and historically the big facts often overshadow the small facts (pace Calder's *Myth of the Blitz*[52]). As a result, accounts that deviate from the overall narrative can be forgotten. This collection of sources however shows that for some, lockdown life offered people the opportunity to learn new skills and to reconnect with family and friends. Some felt that the experience meant that people were 'in this together'. For others the pandemic was divisive, disheartening and disruptive. Their voices, and their experiences, should not be forgotten or lost in the wider narratives that might later emerge.

As seen above, many of the accounts submitted to *#RecordCovid19*, as well as other similar projects, indicate that many people do not believe that their individual experiences are worthy of historical attention, nor do people always recognise that they have lived through moments of history themselves. Since the Second World War, political history and its focus on 'Great Men' has declined in favour of social history and history from below. However, despite the increased attention paid to social history – much of which is public facing – this shift has not quite penetrated the public's perception of what makes history. This disbelief that personal, individual experiences are worthy of historical study seems to be one shared across various cultures and communities. In the case of Britain, where the majority of *#RecordCovid19* responses originated, this belief that history happens to other people is a little strange when one considers that all the respondents lived through Brexit – regardless of one's individual stance on Brexit, it was a profound moment in the social, cultural and political history of Britain and Europe more broadly, and yet the impact on individual lives is often not seen as such.

Historians still have much work to do to convince the public that their experiences will be of historical interest in the future. In an increasingly mediatised age, this is ever more important. The rise of social media platforms such as Twitter, Facebook, Instagram and TikTok, has seen a saturation of artefacts spread across the Internet. Whilst these digital ephemera are often derided today, they will likely be of huge historical interest in the future as they provide us with detailed accounts of the daily lives of people living in the twenty-first century. Perhaps more should be done to assure (or perhaps warn) users of this technology that their lives are historically important and the ephemerality of social media is limited.

The rise of social media has another value to historians. As noted in the Introduction to this collection, *#RecordCovid19* was never intended to be a complete account of the pandemic. It is simply one drop in an ocean of experiences that can only be captured through a range of projects. *#RecordCovid19* and similar projects hopefully demonstrate how a small archive set up by an individual historian relatively

---

52 Angus Calder, *Myth of the Blitz* (London: Pimlico, 2006).

easily can produce a small snapshot of lived experiences as they occur by taking advantage of the plethora of social media that is now available to us. It is the project's intention to build on other accounts from other projects in the future.

History feels like it happens to other people until it happens to us. And Covid-19 happened to us all. We do not know the end of the Covid-19 chapter of history yet. Nor shall we for a long time. Like the staff at the *Yorkshire Evening Post*, many of us would prefer to do without some of the current chapters we find ourselves living through, but as historians, linguists, sociologists, and witnesses to history ourselves, we have to tell these stories. The rest of this collection is an attempt to do just that.

References

Alam, Johnny. 'Transnational Social Media Monuments, Counter-Monuments, and Future of the Nation-State.' In *Monument Culture: International Perspectives on the Future of Monuments in a Changing World*, edited by Laura Macaluso, 191–204. London: Rowman & Littlefield, 2019.

Alexander, Jeffrey C. 'Toward a Theory of Cultural Trauma.' In *Cultural Trauma and Collective Identity*, edited by Jeffrey C. Alexander, Ron Eyerman, Bernard Giesen, Neil J. Smelser, and Piotr Sztompka, 1–30. California: University of California Press, 2004. https://ebookcentral.proquest.com/lib/coventry/detail.action?docID=837285. Accessed 14 April 2023.

Anon. 'Blitz Spirit is Back: Meet The Covid-19 Heroes.' *Daily Telegraph*, 28 March 2020, 5.

Arad Research, 'Collecting Covid Questionnaire 2020: Analysis of Responses: Final Report.' August 2021. https://museum.wales/media/53025/Collecting-Covid-2020_English_Final.pdf. Accessed 13 April 2023.

Calder, Angus. *The Myth of the Blitz*. Pimlico: London, 2006.

Cubitt, Geoffrey. *History and Memory*. Manchester: MUP, 2007.

Davies, Caroline. '"We will Meet Again": Queen Urges Britons To Stay Strong.' *The Guardian*, 5 April 2020, https://www.theguardian.com/world/2020/apr/05/queen-urges-britons-stay-strong-coronavirus-covid-lockdown. Accessed 14 April 2023.

Dudai, Yadin and Micah G. Edelson. 'Personal Memory: Is It Personal, Is It Memory?' *Memory Studies* 9:3 (2016): 275–283. https://doi.org/10.1177/1750698016645234.

Durkheim, Emile. *The Elementary Forms of Religious Life*. London: The Free Press, 1995.

Gessen, Masha. 'The Unimaginable Reality of American Concentration Camps.' *New Yorker*, 21 June 2019. https://www.newyorker.com/news/our-columnists/the-unimaginable-reality-of-american-concentration-camps. Accessed 14 April 2023.

Hoskins, Andrew. 'Flashbulb Memories, Psychology And Media Studies: Fertile Ground For Interdisciplinarity?' *Memory Studies* 2:2 (2009): 147–150. https://doi.org/10.1177/1750698008102049.

Hoskins, Andrew. 'Media, Memory, Metaphor: Remembering and the Connective Turn', *Parallax* 17:4 (2011): 19–31. https://doi.org/10.1080/13534645.2011.605573.

Hoskins, Andrew. 'The Restless Past: An Introduction To Digital Memory And Media.' In *Digital Media Studies*, edited by Andrew Hoskins, 1–24. NY: Taylor and Francis, 2018.

McLuhan, Marshall. *The Gutenberg Galaxy: The Making of Typographic Man*. Toronto: University of Toronto Press, 1962.

Roberts, Sam. 'When History Isn't Something That Happens to Other People.' *New York Times*, 24 April 2002. https://www.nytimes.com/2002/04/24/arts/when-history-isn-t-something-that-happens-to-other-people.html. Accessed 14 April 2023.

Roth, Philip. 'The Story Behind "The Plot Against America."' *The New York Times*, 19 September 2004, 10–12. https://www.nytimes.com/2004/09/19/books/review/the-story-behind-the-plot-against-america.html?smid=url-share. Accessed 14 April 2023.

Schachter, Daniel and Michael Welker. 'Memory And Connection: Remembering The Past And Imagining The Future In Individuals, Groups, And Cultures.' *Memory Studies* 9:3 (2016): 241–244.

Tait, Amelia. 'We Think Of History As Something That Happened To Other People, But We're Living Through It Every Day.' *The New Statesman*, 13 June 2012. https://www.newstatesman.com/politics/uk-politics/2012/06/we-think-history-something-happened-other-people-we-re-living-through-it-every. Accessed 14 April 2023.

Zweig, Stefan. *The World Of Yesterday*. London: Puskin Press, 2009. Kindle Edition.

Online Archives

Lovell, Kristopher. *#RecordCovid19 Project*, https://kristopherlovell.com/category/recordcovid19-project/. Accessed 14 April 2023.

Ward, Michael. *CoronaDiaries: Documenting The Everyday Lived Experiences of a Global Pandemic*. https://collections.swansea.ac.uk/s/coronadiaries/page/home. Accessed 14 April 2023.

Josephine Hoegaerts
Chapter Two
Sounds from A Shrunken World: Covid, Speech and Silence

'My world has shrunk to the space between my house and the corner shop'[1]

Where were you when you experienced your first lockdown? In a bustling Italian city suddenly and brutally brought to a halt? In a remote village where, were it not for the news, you might not have noted the difference? Despite material and contextual differences, quite a number of us reached for the same metaphors to give shape to our experiences for the sudden changes Covid-19 brought to our lives: they 'shrink'.[2] It is an encompassing metaphor, that can cover any number of restrictions to what, until so recently, seemed a 'normal' life. For many, this notion of a shrinking world not only described the restriction of their movements or the sheer space they can inhabit, but also a contraction of the other embodied and lived practices that make up their lives. When one's world shrivels to 'the space between my house and the corner shop', there are fewer people to bump into, fewer places to socialize, and – as this text will concern itself most with – fewer voices to hear. When Covid-19 shrank worlds, it did so materially and spatially but also, I would argue, acoustically: practices of listening and experiences of sound tend to be closely tied to sound's ability to travel, from a mouth to an ear, in intimate gestures or across substantial spatial and emotional divides.[3]

The disruption of these patterns of travelling sound were keenly felt by many – and were even more complicated for atypical ears for whom greater

---

1 [*#RecordCovid19*-80] Female, 28, Awaiting Employment, Wales, https://kristopherlovell.com/2020/09/22/recordcovid19-80-female-28-awaiting-employment-wales/, accessed 21 September 2021.
2 As I will reflect on further on in the text, though, they do not shrink in similar ways or at equal rates depending on one's living circumstances. Several groups of people have had no access to 'remote work' for a variety of reasons, and the rising importance of domesticity likely does not apply to them in the same way.
3 The change to acoustic environments worldwide (and particularly in urban environments) has been reported on extensively. See e.g. Emily Schwing, 'Covid Has Changed Soundscapes Worldwide,' *Scientific American*, 31 May 2020, https://www.scientificamerican.com/podcast/episode/covid-has-changed-soundscapes-worldwide/, accessed 21 September 2021.

Note: Research for this chapter was funded by the European Research Council (ERC StG 2017: CALLIOPE, Vocal Articulations of Parliamentary Identity and Empire)

https://doi.org/10.1515/9783110731002-003

interpersonal distances, headphones, and masks could mean that a 'shrunken' world would become difficult to navigate or even marred by tinnitus. The conflation of lowered mobility, the reduction of (urban) landscapes to all but the most 'essential' services and products, a perceived silencing of the world paired with a sharp rise in domestic demands also seemed to evoke a sense of return to a vague undefined past. This could take a nostalgic turn, as scores of people turned to baking bread, knitting, reading and other activities that seemed to echo rose-tinted views of a former, quieter life.[4] At the same time, feminists warned that the lack of provision of care for children as well as many elderly or disabled family members, and the gendered nature of both domestic and paid care work, risked a 'return to the fifties' for gender politics.[5] The general sense of quiet or silence of lockdown was likewise heard as a 'return' to a less industrially noisy past, with many commenting how they could now hear the birds again, or how the lack of airplane noises reminded them of their childhoods.[6] In a return to both domesticity and nature, it seems, (imaginary) silence reigned.

In this text I want to place the changes to people's soundscapes during the Covid-19 lockdowns in the context of acoustic history and the history of human voices in particular – rather than the quiet, simple domestic pasts that seem to arise so easily in our imagination. I am borrowing the term 'soundscape' from composer

---

4 This is not to say that all those activities are necessarily imagined as either historical or simple. See e.g. Laura Siragusa, 'Reflection: Making Kin with Sourdough During a Pandemic,' *Food and Foodways* 29:1 (2021): 87–96, https://doi.org/10.1080/07409710.2021.1860336.

5 e.g. Heejung Chung, 'Return Of The 1950s Housewife? How To Stop Coronavirus Lockdown Reinforcing Sexist Gender Roles,' *The Conversation*, 30 March 2020, https://theconversation.com/return-of-the-1950s-housewife-how-to-stop-coronavirus-lockdown-reinforcing-sexist-gender-roles-134851, accessed 13 April 2023; Hannah Summers, 'UK society Regressing Back To 1950s For Many Women, Warn Experts,' *The Guardian*, 18 June 2020, https://www.theguardian.com/inequality/2020/jun/18/uk-society-regressing-back-to-1950s-for-many-women-warn-experts-worsening-inequality-lockdown-childcare, accessed 13 April 2023; Emma Jacobs and Laura Noonan, 'Is the Covid-19 Crisis Taking Women Back To The 1950s?' *The Irish Times*, 17 June 2020, https://www.irishtimes.com/business/work/is-the-covid-19-crisis-taking-women-back-to-the-1950s-1.4281579, accessed 13 April 2023.

6 A study of an urban soundscape in the Basque country during lockdown in 2020 shows that these perceived changes to the soundscape were largely shared by different observers, indicating a drop in mechanical sounds (such as cars) in the early phase of lockdown, and a rise in e.g. human and animal sounds heard through open windows. Sara Lenzi, Juan Sádaba, Per Magnus Lindborg, 'Soundscape in Times of Change: Case Study of a City Neighbourhood During the COVID-19 Lockdown,' *Frontiers in Psychology*, March 2021, https://doi.org/10.3389/fpsyg.2021.570741; a study in London shows changes to 'indoor' soundscapes, Simone Torresin et al. 'Indoor Soundscapes At Home During The COVID-19 Lockdown In London – Part I: Associations Between The Perception Of The Acoustic Environment, Occupants' Activity And Well-Being,' *Applied Acoustics* 183 (2021): https://doi.org/10.1016/j.apacoust.2021.108305.

and sound studies scholar Murray Schafer, who conceived of the soundscape as the conglomerate of acoustic features that defined a landscape – not only in terms of its material make-up, but also in relation to its cultural, historical and intersubjective features.[7] The field of 'sound studies', and its sub-field of sound history, has grown exponentially over the last two decades. For this chapter, I mostly rely on approaches that have historically contextualized the mediatized nature of sound, and the effect acoustic practices have on discourses of identity and modernity. For the former, Jonathan Sterne's study of the cultural meaning of acoustic technologies as well as Karin Bijsterveld histories of technological sounds and noises have been formative. For the latter, Holger Schulze's exploration of the sonic persona and Dylan Robinson's critical account of the ethnicized nature of listening are particularly illuminating, as is Daniel Morat's work on the acoustic aspects of 'modern' history.[8]

As historians of sound, like Annelies Jacobs for example, have pointed out, noises and the hum of city sounds are neither modern nor new – the past is only ever imagined as quiet.[9] In doing so, I also include the many mediatized voices that have made up the soundscape of those confined to a shrunken world by looking and listening out of the virtual windows their various screens and audio-devices offer. The text below, first, attempts to sketch aspects of the Covid soundscape, and how it is tied into the historical soundscapes out of which it arose. Rather than trying to offer a representative overview of geopolitical and cultural differences in these soundscapes all over the world[10] I gesture at how such differences are rooted

---

7 R. Murray Schafer, *The Turning of the World* (London: Random House, 1977).

8 Jonathan Sterne, *The Audible Past. Cultural Origins of Sound Reproduction* (Durham: Duke University Press, 2003); Karin Bijsterveld, *Mechanical Sound. Technology, Culture, and Public Problems of Noise in the Twentieth Century* (Boston: MIT Press, 2008); Holger Schulze, *The Sonic Persona. An Anthropology of Sound* (London: Bloomsbury, 2018); Dylan Robinson, *Hungry Listening. Resonant Theory for Indigenous Sound Studies* (Minneapolis: University of Minnesota Press, 2020); Daniel Morat (ed.), *Sounds of Modern History. Auditory Cultures in 19th and 20th century Europe* (New York: Berghahn, 2014) and Josephine Hoegaerts and Kaarina Kilpiö (eds.) 'Sound and Modernity', special collection for *International Journal for History, Culture and Modernity*, 7, (2019).

9 Annelies Jacobs, *Het Geluid Van Gisteren. Waarom Amsterdam Vroeger Ook Niet Stil Was* (Maastricht: Universitaire Pers Maastricht, 2014), 9–11.

10 Numerous projects have sprung up recording narratives, experiences and ideas of life during the pandemic and its lockdowns, which promise to offer opportunities for comparative research in the future. Examples include the Finnish Literature Society, which has a long history of recording personal narratives on different subjects for anthropological and historical research (https://www.finlit.fi/fi/arkisto/vastaa-keruisiin/koronakevat#.YCorijLis2w, accessed 13 April 2023.), the CovidMemory project of the University of Luxembourg (https://covidmemory.lu/, accessed 13 April 2023.) but also attempts to record more specific elements of the pandemic experience, like e.g. the Cities and

in historically grown communities, but also how new audio-visual media have flattened out at least some distinctions. Second, I shift my attention to how these soundscapes have been experienced, and how that experience has been framed as the 'loss' of modern sounds (or sometimes as 'regaining' an imagined auditory past) in the context of work inside and outside the home. The final section of the text reflects on processes of inclusion and exclusion enacted by narratives and practices of listening. Whose experiences of soundscapes, both historical and current, have been made to count? Whose interpretations of stillness and noise have been taken seriously, both historically and now, and who has access to what counts as the salient aspects of the community's soundscape to begin with?

The Silent Conductor – Representations of a New Soundscape

On 17 March 2020, Atso Almila, one of Finland's prime orchestral conductors, tweeted a videoclip of himself on his balcony, conducting part of the Finlandia suite to an invisible orchestra.[11] Invisible and also, as indicated in the tweet's text, inaudible. "Airconducting part of the end of Sibelius' Finlandia (after the hymn), though everyone must imagine the music by themselves. We don't want to disturb anyone", the tweet reads, tagging the popular "Very Finnish Problems" account and therefore suggesting that this quiet approach was intrinsically, if somewhat whimsically, "Finnish". Almila's expert movements were directed at an audience of imaginative listeners, who were called upon to recall Sibelius' iconic music on their own. The video was a response to numerous clips that had been shared on social media from (mostly) China and Italy, where people locked down by the virus had turned to music to rekindle a sense of community – mostly by imagining a history of that community in particular, unified, and consciously stereotypical ways. The conductor's tongue in cheek clip did the same: if the denizens of Wuhan had karaoke, and those of Bergamo could turn to the rich traditions of folk song and opera; the people of Finland had their own national sound: silence.[12] These performances, on

Memory project 'Until We Travel!' which focuses on the changing sounds of mobility and travel: https://citiesandmemory.com/2021/02/open-call-we-need-your-travel-sounds/, accessed 21 Sep 2021.
11 https://twitter.com/soalmila/status/1239904080765558785, accessed 21 September 2021.
12 On (the stereotype of) Finnish silence, see e.g. Eero Tarasti, ed. *Snow, Forest, Silence. The Finnish Tradition of Semiotics*, (Bloomsbury: Indiana University Press, 1999); Pirjo Kukkonen, 'On Silence: The Semiotics of Silence,' in *Acta Semiotica Fennica*, ed. Eero Tarasti (Imatra: International Semiotics Institute, 1993): 283–298; Donal Carbaugh and Saila Poutiainen, 'Silence And Third-

balconies and on social media, were decidedly new, and heavily dependent on hyper-modern technologies, but nevertheless signified something profoundly histori-cal to their performances and audiences. Almila's conducting not only referred to a perceived long history of silence but also to the national romantic music associated with Finland's era of early independence.[13]

Somewhat counterintuitively, perhaps, imagined traditions and historicized practices were used not only to respond to audible changes wrought by life in a pan-demic, but also to consciously craft new sounds. Or, to put it differently, the changing rhythms, locations and limits of life during lockdown changed many ears and the meaning attached to sounds more than they changed the 'actual' soundscape, lead-ing many not only to listen differently, but to produce different sounds too. Some of those practices have been documented in a wide range of reflexions on and analyses of the new soundscapes arising out of lockdown and distancing, as Meri Kytö and Jesse Budel demonstrate in their list of 'Covid 19 Soundscape Resources' for the World Forum of Acoustic Ecology.[14] In March 2020, Cities and Memory launched an appeal to record the sounds of lockdown, #StayHomeSounds, prompting many to contribute with sounds from around the world.[15] Many of the contributions require careful listening, because they record the absence of pre-Covid soundscapes through a focus on silence or quietude in re-discovered natural or muted urban landscapes – such as 'birds on a rainy day in the country', deserted playgrounds or a quiet central market in Ghent where 'the sounds reveal themselves one by one'.[16] That is not to say that the Covid soundscape is only typified by silence – in heavily stricken areas it could be heard as a soundscape of illness and fear, punctuated by the screech of

Party Introductions: An American And Finnish Dialogue,' in *Cultures in Conversation*, ed. Donal Carbaugh (New York: Routledge, 2006), 27–38.

13 Hannu Salmi, 'Jean Sibelius ja Suomalainen kulttuuri- *Finlandian* muuttuvat merkitykset,' in *Sibelius 150: Lahti Sibelius Festival*, eds. Teemu Kirjonen and Taina Räty (Lahti: Sinfonia Lahti, 2015): 12–22.

14 'Covid-19 Soundscape Resources,' https://www.wfae.net/covid-19-soundscapes.html, accessed 13 April 2023.

15 The project explicitly connects acoustic experiences with individual narratives, and stresses the cultural and geo-political specificity of both: contributors upload both a sound recording from their direct environment, and a personal story to go with it. Both are then attached to a map, where listeners can acoustically 'travel' by clicking on different recordings. https://citiesand memory.com/covid19-sounds, accessed 21 Sep 2021.

16 Petri Kuljuntausta, *Schoolyard*, Helsinki, #StayHomeSounds, Stijn Dickel, *The Sounds Reveal Themselves One by One*, Korenmarkt, #StayHomeSounds. It is not surprising, perhaps, that the techniques of listening displayed by contributors to this project seem very close to the ones de-veloped by acoustic ecologist Murray Schafer, who was interested in documenting sound pollu-tion: R. Murray Schafer, *Ear Cleaning. Notes for an Experimental Music Course* (Toronto: Clark and Cruikshank, 1967).

ambulances. The relative quietness of the streets has also turned ears inwards, and not all sounds of domesticity are equally calm and quiet, or indeed peaceful.[17] Additionally, as Sarah Mayberry Scott has pointed out, lockdown also heightened surveillance of numerous (pathologized) sounds produced by bodies confined to domestic or institutional spaces.[18] The silence of lockdown, it seems, is more a social metaphor than an acoustic reality.

What does seem new about the lockdown landscape is how overwhelmingly mediatized it is. Studies of historical (mostly urban) sounds have shown that cities of the past were no quieter than we know them now. In fact, modern ideas about sound pollution may very well have contributed to a relative quietening of the streets.[19] The horse hooves, hawkers, traveling musicians of the early modern and Victorian city have made way for electric cars and terse commuters. Public displays of conflict or joy have become increasingly improper.[20] Conversely, sounds (re)produced by various forms of modern machinery have become much more common in the private sphere – or even in one's private 'bubble' of one.[21] The dominance of such mediatized sounds preceded the arrival of lockdown, but nevertheless seems to have become a salient feature of it. When Walter Ong in 1982 identified the increased reliance on radio, television, telephones and other mediated sound, he probably did not predict the extent to which even personal relations would become

---

17 Police reports in numerous countries have revealed not only higher numbers of domestic violence, but also a rise in disputes between neighbours, the latter of which often based on acoustic disturbance. Historians will be familiar with this practice of listening more closely to the (irritating) sounds of others in quiet environments, such as a library or archive where, as Arlette Farge has famously noted 'slightly laboured breathing becomes conspicuous and agonized wheezing, and a small habit turns into a monstrous tic to be dealt with urgently by psychiatric professionals. In these enclosed spaces, everything is amplified far out of proportion'. Arlette Farge, *The Allure of the Archives* (New Haven: Yale University Press, 2012), 50–51.
18 Sarah Mayberry Scott, 'Sonic Lessons of the Covid-19 Soundscape,' *Sounding Out! blog*, 2 August 2021, https://soundstudiesblog.com/2021/08/02/sonic-lessons-of-the-covid-19-soundscape/, accessed 21 September 2021.
19 As Karin Bijsterveld has shown, the twentieth century is typified mostly by a rise in complaints about noise and a search for silence. Bijsterveld, *Mechanical Sound. Technology, Culture and Public Problems of Noise in the Twentieth Century* (Harvard, MA: MIT Press, 2008), ix, 1–3, 60–64.
20 Not only have noisy traditions like charivaris, public executions, streetfights, etc largely come into increasing disrepute, the modern period also saw a shift from passionate display to 'internalized' emotion, which arguably contributed to a quietening of collectivity. See e.g. Thomas Dixon, *From Passions to Emotions, the Creation of a Secular Psychological Category* (Cambridge: Cambridge University Press, 2003), 135–179.
21 In 1984 already, Shuhei Osawaka introduced the idea of the 'walkman effect'. Hosokawa, 'The Walkman Effect,' *Popular Music* 4 (1984), 165–80.

'virtual'.[22] Ong's schematics of an evolution from orality to literacy to what he called 'secondary orality' has drawn criticism from numerous scholars in literary and sound studies. As, for example, Ivan Kreilkamp and Tom Wright have shown, orality and literacy are not at odds and the expansion of the latter played an important role in supporting the former in the modern period. The spread of print newspapers and novels did not encourage people to quietly stay home and read – it made them talk and read aloud to each other.[23]

Despite such warranted critiques of Ong's framework, I think his attention to different technologies to represent, above all, the spoken word (like writing and recording) plays an important role in how we can understand the changing representation and meanings of sound, and I lean – cautiously – on the broad strokes of his characterization of secondary orality. I also borrow liberally and eclectically from the scholars in sound studies that have questioned and complicated his arguments about the role of audiovisual media in modern life, and wonder how the narratives and sound-files stored in different collections 'work' as recordings. The study of sound recording technology, I would argue, gives us useful clues as to how the practice of recording, both acoustically and in the sense of 'keeping a record', has a cultural meaning of its own, and contributes to our understanding of what we (think we) hear around us.[24] Recent histories of the culture and technology of early recording have shown that, rather than merely 'storing' sound, the act of recording helps to create reality, brings it into being not only in its technological state but also actively helps shape how we speak, sing and sound. People sing (and speak) differently when they know their sounds are being recorded – by machinery, or even by a transcribing human hand.[25]

---

22 Walter Ong, *Orality and Literacy: the Technologizing of the Word* (New York: Methuen, 1982), 133–134.

23 See e.g. Ivan Kreilkamp, *Voice and the Victorian Storyteller* (Cambridge: Cambridge University Press, 2005), 2–3; Tom F. Wright, 'Proclaiming the War News: Richard Caton Woodville and Herman Melville,' in *War and Literature*, eds. Laura Ashe and Ian Patterson (Cambridge: D.S. Brewer, 2014), 163–182.

24 On the practice of recording and its work across different media, see e.g. Lisa Gitelman, *Paper Media: Toward a Media History of Documents* (Durham: Duke University Press, 2014); *Scripts, Grooves and Writing Machines: Representing Technology in the Edison Era* (Redwood City, CA: Stanford University Press, 2000); Nicholas Cook, *Beyond the Score. Music as Performance* (Oxford: Oxford University Press, 2013); Delphine Gardey, *Écrire, Calculer, Classer. Comment Une Révolution De Papier A Transformé Les Sociétés Contemporaines (1800–1940)* (Paris: La Découverte, 2008).

25 On the influence of recording technology on vocal technique, see Karin Martensen, »*The phonograph is not an opera house*«.: *Quellen und Analysen zu Ästhetik und Geschichte der frühen Tonaufnahme am Beispiel von Edison und Victor* (Munich: Allitera Verlag, 2019); 21–24 on the 'phonographic' qualities of transcription, see e.g. John Picker, *Victorian Soundscapes* (Oxford: Oxford University Press, 2003), 133–141.

In a world of virtual communication in which we rely on audio-visual technology for news, entertainment and personal interaction, it is not only the voices of opera singers and politicians that are co-created by technology. We have all become carriers of mediatized sound. The contributions to various projects recording stories, memories, and sounds of Covid 19 also show struggles with that change.[26]

The Neighbour Who Won't Stop Mowing his Lawn – Experiences of the Lockdown Soundscape

Efforts to record the experience of lockdown and life during the pandemic, although often focusing on doing and feeling, contain a number of clues about the audible world of contributors. #StayHomeSounds does so most consistently but – in its focus on recorded sound – perhaps least explicitly. Searching through the collection allows one to dive into the soundscape of Covid around the world, with a map giving an explicitly 'spatial' feel to all the recordings and suggesting the possibility to immerse oneself, acoustically, in different environments. But in textual records, too, witnesses have commented on their experience of what could perhaps be called a Covid soundscape. A soundscape that, for some at least, seems to be mostly characterized by loss or, as one person expressed it, 'the absence of the rumble of normality'.[27] It is an absence that implies a very particular kind of silence – not simply the absence, or reduced presence, of sound, but the absence of a noise mostly associated with city life. Similarly, another witness notes the sudden audibility of birds chirping.[28] The world, it seems, has turned into a bucolic postcard. The sounds so strongly associated with the franticness and technology of modern life seem out of place in such a soundscape and the ring of telephones therefore appears both as a lifeline connecting to 'normality' and a disruption to the seemingly peaceful soundscape of daily life. Several contributions note how the phone has become a more important and more noticeable presence.[29]

---

26 In this text, I am mostly relying on the collections of *#RecordCovid19* (https://kristopherlovell.com/category/record-covid-19-project/, accessed 21 September 2021.) and #StayHomeSounds (https://citiesandmemory.com/covid19-sounds/).

27 [*#RecordCovid19*-9] Bridgnorth, Bar Manager, Male, 25,https://kristopherlovell.com/2020/04/16/record-covid19-9-bridgnorth-bar-manager-male-25/, accessed 21 September 2021.

28 [*#RecordCovid19*-33] Turkey, Student, Male, 25, https://kristopherlovell.com/2020/04/27/record-covid19-33-turkey-student-male-25/, accessed 21 September 2021.

29 See for example: [*#RecordCovid19*-23] West Wales, Freelance Teacher, Trainer, Project Manager, Female. 61, https://kristopherlovell.com/2020/04/24/record-covid19-23-west-wales-freelance-teacher-trainer-project-manager-female-61/, accessed 21 September 2021; [*#RecordCovid19*-44],

Other signs of mechanic sound are even more disruptive. 'My neighbour won't stop mowing the lawn', one young woman writes. 'I think, therefore I am. I hear the constant roar of a lawnmower, therefore I am irritated. I didn't know it was possible for one man to mow the lawn so often. I'm amazed that he has any lawn left'.[30] Such noises do not only pierce the quietude people connect to lockdown, but they also undermine the metaphoric silence that isolation seems to be associated with. As days become less marked by collective performances of busyness, the soundscape seems to have taken on a repetitive quality that is culturally understood as quiet not because it lacks sound, but because it lacks the specific sounds we have learned to hear as 'modern' and industrious. The relative lack of intersubjective vocal interaction contributes to this sense of repetitiveness and quietude. Centuries of elevating the sound of a human voice above all others, in meaningfulness, expressivity and even beauty, have attuned our ears to its timbres and melodies. Being cut off from direct spoken interaction – even if only by a screen – is perhaps exacerbated by the enormous vocabularies most cultures have developed about the importance of speech in human interaction.[31]

And yet, despite a keenly felt lack of human voices, we live our lives surrounded by them. They come to us from various screens, out of the earplugs we carry around as we furtively go for our weekly grocery trips. Most of us can recite some salient sound bite recently uttered by public political figures ('I felt it was a pandemic long before it was called a pandemic'), and we hear their voices in our collective and individual imaginations. So suffused with the political spoken word is our world, that we even hear their absence as silence. When Angela Merkel prepared to go into quarantine, early in 2020, we collectively felt the disappearance of her voice even before it happened.[32] When Boris Johnson landed in hospital, we learned that in the face of vocal political silence, the simple act of breathing can take centre stage and

---

Student, 21, Female, https://kristopherlovell.com/2020/05/04/record-covid19-44-student-21-female/, accessed 21 September 2021.

30 [*#RecordCovid19*-27] UK, Unemployed (the current national occupation), Female, 27, https://kristopherlovell.com/2020/04/25/record-covid19-27-uk-unemployed-the-current-national-occupation-female-27/, accessed 21 September 2021.

31 The notion that speech is what 'makes us human' goes back to ancient Greece, at least, and has continued to rear its head throughout history, including in ableist and psychological iterations (think, for example, of the insistence on oralist education for Deaf children, or more recent beliefs about the power of 'talking to someone' to preserve one's mental health). Joanna Bourke, *What it Means to be Human* (London: Virago Press, 2013), part I; John Heath, *The Talking Greeks* (Cambridge: Cambridge University Press, 2005).

32 'Kanzlerin Merkel in häuslicher Quarantäne,' *Der Spiegel,* 22 March 2020, https://www.spiegel.de/politik/deutschland/coronakrise-kanzlerin-merkel-in-haeuslicher-quarantaene-a-bcde5f71-4c0e-468d-ae28-bce71dc5a9e8, accessed 21 September 2021.

become a public message.[33] The collection of *#RecordCovid19*, with its wealth of British experiences, is punctuated by the appearances of the prime minister. One young man noted how these appearances ruptured domestic acoustic spaces: 'Those 4 or 5 minutes of absolute silence, save the television' denoting a sense of importance.[34]

This universe in which whole nations can be found listening out anxiously for the breathing rhythms of their public figures as well as their loved ones, seems to have arisen in an instant. It was created by a sudden crisis and supported by modern audio-visual technology. We hear Macron's voice in our heads, we think, because we also hear him coming out of our digital devices so often. We can imitate Trudeau 'speaking moistly' because we live in an age of sound bites, aural memes and TikTok videos.[35] Amid the new fears around a spreading pandemic, ongoing tensions between social and traditional media rage on, with journalists despairing of the preponderance of the sound bite and clickbait, insisting that the long read, the in-depth interview, are not only more informative or correct (and thus 'superior'), but also that they are more solid gateways to knowledge because of their connections to traditions of the craft, that their older historical pedigree matters and sets them apart from faddish obsessions with the sound bite.

The stream of misinformation, badly referenced graphs, shaky scientific premises and just plain 'fake news' is denounced as part of this new phenomenon and a (direct) result of a new media culture that has been embraced wholeheartedly by populist movements and progressive politicians alike. But populism is hardly new – and neither, I would argue, is the sound-bite. Victorian newspapers are full of sharp witticisms – Oscar Wilde was a well-known master of the genre, but he was certainly not alone. These look more like 'literature' to us now, because we only ever encounter them in the written form, but they had a distinctly oral origin, and retained that flavour for their contemporary readers, much in the way we can 'hear' Trump's tweets in his voice when we read them. More importantly, perhaps, the tone employed by numerous public figures whose voices surround us now, has

---

33 As shown by the particular attention given to the question of whether the prime minister would need a ventilator. See e.g. 'Boris Johnson: it was 50–50 whether to put me on a ventilator,' *The Guardian*, 3 May 2020, https://www.theguardian.com/world/2020/may/03/boris-johnson-it-was-50-50-whether-to-put-me-on-ventilator-coronavirus, accessed 21 September 2021; Christina Gallardo, 'Reports Boris Johnson Is On A Ventilator Are 'Russian Disinformation,'' *Politico*, 6 April 2020, https://www.politico.eu/article/reports-boris-johnson-is-on-a-ventilator-are-russian-disinformation/, accessed 21 September 2021.

34 [*#RecordCovid19*-39] Lincolnshire, Accountant, Male, 23, https://kristopherlovell.com/2020/04/28/record-covid19-38-lincolnshire-accountant-male-23/, accessed 21 September 2021.

35 Anonymotif (Brock Tyler), *Speaking Moistly*, YouTube, 2020, https://www.youtube.com/watch?v=eySDeBdqxGY, accessed 21 September 2021.

arisen from long-standing political and educational traditions: those of teaching young elites how to speak in public.

The almost obsessive focus on the news and on central public figures many report – whilst having found new expressions – is therefore deeply rooted in the history of representative democracy. The authority of not only the spoken word in general, but the practice of standing up and speaking out loud as a means of political representation seems to have lost little of its power, even in the increasingly virtual world of lockdown. Listeners express their exasperation at the use of 'pre-recorded speeches' which seem to be heard as less authentic or real than 'live' performances.[36] Others, in criticizing the reliance on prepared speeches or politicians' excessive 'words' echo the irritation with practices of representative democracy that can be traced back to the nineteenth century, when observers already criticized the fact that 'the gift of the gab' could trump intelligence.[37] For all our increased comfort with the heightened mediatization of sound, we still seem to distrust the politician who aims his speeches at the scribblers' gallery rather than his peers and constituents.[38]

The Lady Who Lived in a Book – Whose Ears Make the Soundscape?

The perception and experience of the Covid soundscape as one characterized by silences reminiscent of a less technological and more tranquil past rely, as the previous sections suggest, on a number of cultural scripts inherited from historical discourses about life, domesticity and democracy. The various inequalities that have fed into those scripts, historically, largely seem to shine through in experiences of the Covid soundscape as well. Images of cosily staying in likely have little real meaning for single mothers trapped with boisterous children in a small apartment; the bustle of the modern city may hold little attraction if its streets are inaccessible to you and your wheelchair, and the equation of political authority and

---

36 [*#RecordCovid19*-52] London, Civil Servant, 25–30, https://kristopherlovell.com/2020/05/11/recordcovid19-52-london-civil-servant-25-30/, accessed 21 September 2021.
37 [*#RecordCovid19*-18] Wales, Writer, Female, 27, https://kristopherlovell.com/2020/04/23/record-covid-19-18-wales-writer-female-27/, accessed 21 September 2021; [*#RecordCovid*19-53] W. Wales, Freelance Teacher, Trainer, Project Manager, Female. 61, https://kristopherlovell.com/2020/05/11/recordcovid19-53-w-wales-freelance-teacher-trainer-project-manager-female-61/, accessed 21 September 2021; Benjamin Beasley, *Reminiscences of a Stammerer,* (London: The Roxburghe Press, 1902), 123.
38 Andrew Sparrow, *Obscure Scribblers: A History of Parliamentary Journalism* (London: Politicos, 2003), 153–155.

representation with 'good speech' excludes anyone who does not speak or hear with ease. As has been pointed out by numerous commentators, the exceptionalism of lockdown and its experience has largely been presented and lived as the experience not only of the able-bodied western heteronormative double income couple, but also as decidedly middle class.[39] Therefore, in this final section, I want to turn a more critical and more consciously diversity-seeking ear to what I have been calling the Covid soundscape, and wonder whose ears we are taking seriously, when we think about the sounds of lockdown as a characteristic component of pandemic life.

The sounds recorded in collections like *#RecordCovid19* and #StayHomeSounds, I would argue, present not only a limited but also a somewhat scripted version of what the pandemic has sounded like. Some of that scripted quality is guided by the instructions and focus of the collections themselves, some is probably the result of witnesses being self-selected (i.e. those with the kind of literacy to find the call and the leisure time to engage with them as well as the skills and technology required to write a narrative or curate and record sounds). As a result, the reports seem to privilege the experiences of mostly able bodied adults, with little or no mobility issues and largely in knowledge-based jobs.[40] For that section of the population, the imagined tranquillity of lockdown co-exists with the ubiquity of new audiovisual technology as they spend the day catching up with family on the phone, despairing over having to date over video chat or getting exasperated by an endless day of staring at screens and trying to 'manage their tone' as they adapt to new forms in communication in both their professional and private lives.[41] Despite some enthusiasm over this technology ('thank god for video calling!'),[42] the rapid increase of many employees'

---

39 e.g. Lynsey Hanley, 'Lockdown Has Laid Bare British Class Divide,' *The Guardian*, 7 April 2020, https://www.theguardian.com/commentisfree/2020/apr/07/lockdown-britain-victorian-class-divide, accessed 21 September 2021. As a counternarrative, Lisa Mackenzie's project on working class lockdown diaries offers a different perspective. Mackenzie, '"It's Only 11am And Everyone Is Crying": Working-Class Diaries Of Lockdown,' *LSE Covid 19 Blog*, 19 April 2021, https://blogs.lse. ac.uk/covid19/2021/04/19/its-only-11am-and-everyone-is-crying-working-class-diaries-of-lockdown/, accessed 21 September 2021.

40 It is perhaps important to note that a sizeable minority designated themselves as unemployed, too, some commenting on the effects of the pandemic on the availability of work.

41 [*#RecordCovid19*-16], London, Civil Servant, Female, 25, https://kristopherlovell.com/2020/04/21/record-covid-19-16-london-female-25-civil-servant/, accessed 21 September 2021; [*#RecordCovid19*-15] Wales, Engineer, Female, 30, https://kristopherlovell.com/2020/04/21/record-covid-19-15-wales-engineer-female-30/, Accessed 21 September 2021.

42 [*#RecordCovid19*-17]. North West UK, Sales Rep, Female 57 yrs old, https://kristopherlovell.com/2020/04/22/record-covid-19-17north-west-uk-sales-rep-female-57-yrs-old/, accessed 21 September 2021.

dependency on new technologies and machines generates anxiety too – one reminiscent of the anxieties that surrounded the birth of the modern office.[43]

Machines have, historically, had a habit of making workers nervous and insecure – often with good reason, as machines, along with reducing the need for heavy physical labour, tend to also lead to a loss of respect for skilled labour, higher standards for productivity and (thus) comparatively longer hours, lower wages and more repetitive work.[44] They also tend to facilitate changes to the workforce itself – both the industrial revolution and the arrival of the telephone and typewriter created a place for (single) women to take up regular non-domestic work, for example.[45] The rapid rise of video-calling, chat and other forms of remote communication (not all of them dependent on the capacity to take part in spoken conversation) could perhaps, similarly, open up possibilities for new definitions of what constitutes work. Or more importantly, it might disrupt existing narratives about who is considered fit to work, and shake up pre-conceived notions about which characteristics support good leadership, or good communication at work – particularly in office environments. As historians of bureaucracy and office management have pointed out, the 'invention' of the quiet and efficient office in the late nineteenth century was connected to very specific understandings of workplace hierarchies, enacted through space and articulated in the soundscape.[46] With both those spaces and their soundscapes no longer a given, the 'office' may very well enact new inclusions and exclusions at work. The reliance on technologies like videocalling and its (imperfect) possibilities for captioning opens up avenues for workers with limited mobility, for example, but also interacts differently with different types of hearing and deafness. One contributor to *#RecordCovid19* reported how a rise in tinnitus interfered with their concentration.[47]

Modern office culture had long been based on older understandings of middle class norms surrounding speech and silence. In performances of middle class

43 Delphine Gardey, *La Dactylographe Et L'expeditionnaire: Histoire Des Employes De Bureau, 1890–1930* (Paris: Belin, 2001), 127–135.

44 See e.g. Tim Cresswell, *On the Move* (New York: Routledge, 2006), 85–122.

45 The influence of such technologies is culturally specific as well, as Kerim Yasar's history of the cultural influence and meaning of the telephone in Japan shows. Kerim Yasar, *Electrified Voices. How the Telephone, Phonograph and Radio Shaped Modern Japan 1868–1945* (New York: Columbia University Press, 2018).

46 Jens Van De Maele, 'From Bentham To Guadet: "Auditory Visibility" In Nineteenth-Century Theories On Government Offices,' *International Journal for History, Culture and Modernity* 7:1 (2019): 673–685.

47 [*#RecordCovid19*-25], Berlin, Student, Genderqueer, 25, https://kristopherlovell.com/2020/04/24/record-covid19-25-berlin-student-genderqueer-25/, accessed 21 September 2021.

(male) identity, both silence and speech, if done well, signalled authority and independence.[48] Freedom from the clatter of the street as well as the capacity to avoid idle chatter. Freedom from the kind of situations and institutions where speech could be extracted, like schools or mental institutions, as well as a trained and modulated voice for public speech. In such a cultural system, a balance between authoritative speech and calm silence represented a privileged norm, while other types of speech or silences were heard as less dignified, and often pathologized.[49] Despite considerable changes to public and private life, the pandemic soundscape seems to have revived some of the tensions connected to silence and speech in new ways. Once again, quiet and stillness is a sign of privilege for some – those who can retreat to a domestic world of relative calm – and a sign of pathology for others – those who struggle with loneliness, or those who cannot quite get the hang of new audio-visual technology.

The stark differences in how speech and silence have been distributed within the covid-soundscape, together with this renewed tension between privileged and pathologized silences, all work to strengthen the sense that pandemic life presents a return to the past too. Not (only) to a bucolic world of nature and domesticity, but also to a world in which the model of domesticity held up as the norm is that of a middle class heterosexual household, provided for by an adult man and held together by the 'angel of the house'. It has been observed repeatedly that the pandemic – including lockdowns – has had an outsized impact on women, who carry most of the burden of both unpaid and paid care-work. I would argue, however, that at least in theory the pandemic also presents opportunities to radically rethink work, domesticity and the relationship between them. The middle-class breadwinner model, both in its nineteenth-century inception and in its iconic 1950's reiteration, was based on a separation between the home and the office, between the domestic and the public realms – with women largely confined to the home, and men travelling between the private and public world.[50] This model, which was

---

48 Josephine Hoegaerts, 'Speaking Like Intelligent Men: Vocal Articulations of Authority and Identity in the House of Commons in the Nineteenth Century,' *Radical History Review*, 121 (2015): 123–144.

49 On the multiplicity of silence, and its different guises at the crossroads with social difference and identity, see e.g. Josephine Hoegaerts and Pieter Verstraete, *Silence and Diversity*, special issue DiGest, 2016.

50 On the ideals of gendered domesticity and the fiction of 'separate spheres', see e.g. John Tosh, *A Man's Place. Masculinity and the Middle Class Home in Victorian England* (New Haven: Yale University Press, 1999), 53–79; Amanda Vickery, 'Golden Age To Separate Spheres? A Review Of The Categories And Chronology Of English Women's History,' *Historical Journal* 36, (1993): 383–414. This model of the nuclear family also ignores the large numbers of unmarried women involved in informal and formal childcare throughout history (as nurses, aunts, nuns, teachers, etc).

always myth more than a reality, has come under pressure in the last half century in a variety of ways. The current conflation of home and work, for the middle classes at least, creates a new kind of pressure again. The confusing, counterintuitive soundscape of lockdown is one articulation of that pressure, and one we have, perhaps, not quite learned how to hear.

*

Speaking about a 'lockdown soundscape' or a soundscape of the pandemic is a risky business. There is, of course, no one soundscape to be heard, dependent as it is on environment, human and non-human practices, and especially embodied and encultured ears. Nevertheless, two things about the impact of the pandemic and its lockdowns on the acoustic environment seem clear. First, the changes of the rhythm and organization of life have brought changes to various sounding environments. And second, the way we make sense of those changes in acoustic environments are highly marked by historically defined cultural scripts. While our ears are all culturally, socially and individually different, we share the habit of depending on the past to make sense of what we hear in the present.[51] And thus, 'pre recorded speeches' leave us imagining a less trustworthy practice of speech than live debate. Or we imagine 'silence' to accompany the feeling of a shrinking world despite the din of delivery vans, sirens and televisions. Especially when it comes to the sounds of lockdown, our ears and cultural expressions cling stubbornly to a form of domesticity that sits uneasily with the reality of remote work, the redomestication of carework and the relentless noise of mediatized politics and entertainment. As witnesses in *#RecordCovid19* struggle to express, the space their world has shrunken into is not necessarily their house, or the bucolic image of a cottage in a village with a cornerstore. The new soundscape is a mediatized and largely 'loud' one that gains meaning as listeners make sense of it. For some it is 'like being in a sci-fi film', for others it's a 'horror movie', and for at least one person, it felt like being 'in a book'.[52] That last image, particularly, opens up possibilities to rethink our own agency within the limited confines of lockdown life, and perhaps might even encourage us, now that many of the norms and expectations of 'modern' life have been upended, to turn a couple of pages. At the very least,

---

51 This has been termed the 'period ear', experiences and practices of listening are historically defined and change over time.

52 [*#RecordCovid19*-39] Lincolnshire, Accountant, Male, 23, https://kristopherlovell.com/2020/04/28/re cord-covid19-38-lincolnshire-accountant-male-23/, accessed 21 September 2021; [*#RecordCovid19*-38] Turkey, Student, Female, 18, https://kristopherlovell.com/2020/04/28/record-covid19-37-turkey-stu dent-female-18/, accessed 21 September 2021; [*#RecordCovid19*-1], Croydon, Civil Servant, Female, 25, https://kristopherlovell.com/2020/04/12/record-covid-19-1-croydon-civil-servant-female-25/, accessed 21 September 2021.

the various attempts to capture and somehow 'record' soundscapes of lockdown life can alert us to the importance we attach to our sounding environments, and to the multiple methods that can be used to make such recordings. The narrative, often almost poetic quality, of many reflections on the acoustic changes wrought by covid call the assumed objectivity, accuracy, and completeness of acoustic recording into question, and suggest that in order to think through soundscapes historically, we need to look beyond ambitions of 'hi-fi' solutions to storing sound.[53] Historians of sound, with their experience of interpreting the manifold expressions of acoustic experiences and meanings through other, non-sounding, media, can therefore offer vantagepoints from which to re-interpret soundscapes of change and of crisis that go beyond metaphors of 'listening' to historical actors, and delve into the cultural and political meaning of crisis narratives.

References

Anon. 'Kanzlerin Merkel in häuslicher Quarantäne.' *Der Spiegel*, 22 March 2020. https://www.spiegel.de/politik/deutschland/coronakrise-kanzlerin-merkel-in-haeuslicher-quarantaene-a-bcde5f71-4c0e-468d-ae28-bce71dc5a9e8. Accessed 21 September 2021.

Anonymotif (Brock Tyler). *Speaking Moistly*. YouTube, 2020. https://www.youtube.com/watch?v=eySDeBdqxGY. Accessed 21 September 2021.

Beasley, Benjamin. *Reminiscences of a Stammerer*. London: The Roxburghe Press, 1902.

Bijsterveld, Karin. *Mechanical Sound. Technology, Culture, and Public Problems of Noise in the Twentieth Century*. Boston: MIT Press, 2008.

Bourke, Joanna. *What it Means to be Human*. London: Virago Press, 2013.

Carbaugh, Donal and Saila Poutiainen. 'Silence And Third-Party Introductions: An American And Finnish Dialogue.' In *Cultures in Conversation*, edited by Donal Carbaugh, 27–38. New York: Routledge, 2006.

Chung, Heejung. 'Return Of The 1950s Housewife? How To Stop Coronavirus Lockdown Reinforcing Sexist Gender Roles.' *The Conversation*, 30 March 2020. https://theconversation.com/return-of-the-1950s-housewife-how-to-stop-coronavirus-lockdown-reinforcing-sexist-gender-roles-134851. Accessed 21 September 2021.

Cook, Nicholas. *Beyond the Score. Music as Performance*. Oxford: Oxford University Press, 2013.

Cresswell, Tim. *On the Move*. New York: Routledge, 2006.

Dixon, Thomas, *From Passions to Emotions, the Creation of a Secular Psychological Category*. Cambridge: Cambridge University Press, 2003.

Farge, Arlette. *The Allure of the Archives*. New Haven: Yale University Press, 2012.

---

53 On the difficult relationship between the passing of time and recording technology, as well as the recurring dream of accurate acoustic recording, see e.g. Melle Kromhout, 'Hearing Pastness And Presence: The Myth Of Perfect Fidelity And The Temporality Of Recorded Sound,' *Sound Studies: an Interdisciplinary Journal* 6:1 (2020): 29–44.

Gallardo, Christina. 'Reports Boris Johnson is on a ventilator are "Russian disinformation."' *Politico*, 6 April 2020. https://www.politico.eu/article/reports-boris-johnson-is-on-a-ventilator-are-russian-disinformation/. Accessed 21 September 2021.

Gardey, Delphine. *Écrire, Calculer, Classer. Comment Une Révolution De Papier A Transformé Les Sociétés Contemporaines (1800–1940)* Paris: La Découverte, 2008.

Gardey, Delphine. *La Dactylographe Et L'expeditionnaire: Histoire Des Employes De Bureau, 1890–1930*. Paris: Belin, 2001.

Gitelman, Lisa. *Paper Media: Toward a Media History of Documents*. Durham: Duke University Press, 2014.

Gitelman, Lisa. *Scripts, Grooves and Writing Machines: Representing Technology in the Edison Era*. Redwood City, CA: Stanford University Press, 2000.

Hanley, Lynsey. "Lockdown has laid bare British class divide." *The Guardian*, 7 April 2020. https://www.theguardian.com/commentisfree/2020/apr/07/lockdown-britain-victorian-class-divide. Accessed 21 September 2021.

Heath, John. *The Talking Greeks*. Cambridge: Cambridge University Press, 2005.

Hoegaerts, Josephine and Kaarina Kilpiö (eds.). 'Sound and Modernity' special collection for *International Journal for History, Culture and Modernity* 7 (2019).

Hoegaerts, Josephine and Pieter Verstraete. *Silence and Diversity*, special issue DiGest, 2016.

Hoegaerts, Josephine. 'Speaking Like Intelligent Men: Vocal Articulations of Authority and Identity in the House of Commons in the Nineteenth Century.' *Radical History Review* 121 (2015): 123–144.

Hosokawa, Shuhei. 'The Walkman Effect.' *Popular Music* 4 (1984): 165–180.

Jacobs, Annelies. *Het Geluid Van Gisteren. Waarom Amsterdam Vroeger Ook Niet Stil Was*. Maastricht: Universitaire Pers Maastricht, 2014.

Jacobs, Emma and Laura Noonan. 'Is The Covid-19 Crisis Taking Women Back To The 1950s?' *The Irish Times*, 17 June 2020. https://www.irishtimes.com/business/work/is-the-covid-19-crisis-taking-women-back-to-the-1950s-1.4281579. Accessed 21 September 2021.

Kreilkamp, Ivan. *Voice and the Victorian Storyteller*. Cambridge: Cambridge University Press, 2005.

Kromhout, Melle. 'Hearing Pastness And Presence: The Myth Of Perfect Fidelity And The Temporality Of Recorded Sound.' *Sound Studies: an Interdisciplinary Journal* 6:1 (2020): 29–44.

Kukkonen, Pirjo. 'On Silence: the Semiotics of Silence.' In *Acta Semiotica Fennica*, edited by Eero Imatra Tarasti. International Semiotics Institute, 1993.

Lenzi, Sara., Juan Sádaba and Per Magnus Lindborg. 'Soundscape in Times of Change: Case Study of a City Neighbourhood During the COVID-19 Lockdown.' *Frontiers in Psychology*, March 2021. https://doi.org/10.3389/fpsyg.2021.570741.

Mackenzie, Lisa. '"It's Only 11am And Everyone Is Crying": Working-Class Diaries Of Lockdown.' *LSE Covid 19 Blog*, 19 April 2021. https://blogs.lse.ac.uk/covid19/2021/04/19/its-only-11am-and-everyone-is-crying-working-class-diaries-of-lockdown/. Accessed 21 September 2021.

Martensen, Karin. *»The phonograph is not an opera house«.: Quellen und Analysen zu Ästhetik und Geschichte der frühen Tonaufnahme am Beispiel von Edison und Victor*. Munich: Allitera Verlag, 2019.

Mayberry Scott, Sarah. 'Sonic Lessons of the Covid-19 Soundscape.' *Sounding Out! blog*, 2 August 2021. https://soundstudiesblog.com/2021/08/02/sonic-lessons-of-the-covid-19-soundscape/. Accessed 21 September 2021.

Morat, Daniel (ed.). *Sounds of Modern History. Auditory Cultures in 19th and 20th century Europe*. New York: Berghahn, 2014.

Ong, Walter. *Orality and Literacy: the Technologizing of the Word*. New York: Methuen, 1982.

Picker, John. *Victorian Soundscapes*. Oxford: Oxford University Press, 2003.

Proctor, Kate and Nazia Parveen. 'Boris Johnson: it was 50-50 whether to put me on a ventilator.' *The Guardian*, 3 May 2020. https://www.theguardian.com/world/2020/may/03/boris-johnson-it-was-50-50-whether-to-put-me-on-ventilator-coronavirus. Accessed 21 September 2021.

Robinson, Dylan. *Hungry Listening. Resonant Theory for Indigenous Sound Studies*, Minneapolis: University of Minnesota Press, 2020.

Salmi, Hannu. 'Jean Sibelius ja Suomalainen kulttuuri- *Finlandian* muuttuvat merkitykset.' In *Sibelius 150: Lahti Sibelius Festival*, eds. Teemu Kirjonen and Taina Räty, 12–22. Lahti: Sinfonia Lahti, 2015.

Schafer, R. Murray. *Ear Cleaning. Notes for an Experimental Music Course*. Toronto: Clark & Cruikshank, 1967.

Schafer, R. Murray. *The Turning of the World*. London: Random House, 1977.

Schulze, Holger. *The Sonic Persona. An Anthropology of Sound*. London: Bloomsbury, 2018.

Schwing, Emily. 'Covid Has Changed Soundscapes Worldwide.' *Scientific American*, 31 May 2020, https://www.scientificamerican.com/podcast/episode/covid-has-changed-soundscapes-worldwide/. Accessed 21 September 2021.

Siragusa, Laura. 'Reflection: Making Kin with Sourdough During a Pandemic.' *Food and Foodways* 29:1 (2021). https://doi.org/10.1080/07409710.2021.1860336.

Sparrow, Andrew. *Obscure Scribblers: A History of Parliamentary Journalism*, London: Politicos, 2003.

Sterne, Jonathan. *The Audible Past. Cultural Origins of Sound Reproduction*, Durham: Duke University Press, 2003.

Summers, Hannah. 'UK Society Regressing Back To 1950s For Many Women, Warn Experts.' *The Guardian*, 18 June 2020, https://www.theguardian.com/inequality/2020/jun/18/uk-society-regressing-back-to-1950s-for-many-women-warn-experts-worsening-inequality-lockdown-childcare. Accessed 21 September 2021.

Tarasti, Eero (ed.). *Snow, Forest, Silence. The Finnish Tradition of Semiotics*. Bloomsbury: Indiana University Press, 1999.

Torresin, Simone., Rossano Albatici, Francesco Aletta, Francesco Babich, Tin Oberman, Agnieszka Elzbieta Stawinoga and Jian Kang. 'Indoor Soundscapes At Home During The COVID-19 Lockdown In London – Part I: Associations Between The Perception Of The Acoustic Environment, Occupants' Activity And Well-Being.' *Applied Acoustics* 183, 2021, https://doi.org/10.1016/j.apacoust.2021.108305.

Tosh, John. *A Man's Place. Masculinity and the Middle Class Home in Victorian England*. New Haven: Yale University Press, 1999.

Van De Maele, Jens. 'From Bentham To Guadet: "Auditory Visibility" In Nineteenth-Century Theories On Government Offices.' *International Journal for History, Culture and Modernity* (2019): 673–685.

Vickery, Amanda. 'Golden Age To Separate Spheres? A Review Of The Categories And Chronology Of English Women's History', *Historical Journal* 36 (1993): 383–414.

Wright, Tom F. 'Proclaiming the War News: Richard Caton Woodville and Herman Melville.' In *War and Literature*, eds. Laura Ashe and Ian Patterson, 163–182. Cambridge: D.S. Brewer, 2014.

Yasar, Kerim. *Electrified Voices. How the Telephone, Phonograph and Radio Shaped Modern Japan 1868–1945*. New York: Columbia University Press, 2018.

Elizabeth Benjamin and Sarah Turner

Chapter Three
Pregnancy and Parenthood through the Covid Pandemic: Changing Pressures and Priorities

The journey to parenthood is one that even at the best of times is filled with hope, but also with fear; despite advances in prenatal screening and neonatal healthcare, pregnancy and birth carries risks to baby and parent alike, and there remains a degree of uncertainty around the outcome of the process. The pandemic took this experience into new realms of the unknown. The novel coronavirus, which became a pandemic in March 2020 and led to the imposition of varying degrees of restrictions worldwide in an attempt to curtail its spread, brought a set of particular challenges to the experience of pregnancy and birth.

Some of the challenges faced by pregnant individuals[1] throughout the pandemic were exacerbated by a (perhaps unique) conflict inherent in the areas of pregnancy and childbirth between the 'medical' and the 'personal'; a pregnant person receives medical care and is considered a 'patient', but is not inherently unwell. Decision-making throughout the process hinges on this binary: a parent is an expert in their own preferences, but is usually not a doctor; a doctor is a medical expert, but cannot make decisions for the patient, except in cases where a patient lacks the capacity to do so.[2] The pandemic added further complexity to this dynamic, by demanding that the 'personal' be pared back in favour of the safety of the community. The contentious intersections between the medical and the personal were further complicated in regard to accompanying partners. While pregnancy and birth are medical(ised) procedures, they are also unique in that it is expected that the 'patient' will be accompanied by a (non-medical) partner, friend, or supporter. Tightening restrictions forced many people to attend prenatal appointments and to give birth alone, as personal choice was curtailed by the need to ensure public safety.

---

1 Throughout this chapter we have used gender neutral terminology for the purposes of inclusivity. We recognise that while the experience of pregnancy and birth is restricted to individuals who are biologically female, this does not mean that those who undergo it identify as women. We would like to avoid any binary oppositions in this regard and promote inclusivity as far as possible.
2 General Medical Council, 'Decision Making and Consent,' https://www.gmc-uk.org/ethical-guidance/ethical-guidance-for-doctors/decision-making-and-consent, accessed 12 January 2023.

https://doi.org/10.1515/9783110731002-004

Even where a choice was available, the pandemic brought new factors to these choices. Expectant parents had to make decisions around their birth options while taking into account their risk of infection, as well as the inherent risks of pregnancy; while a homebirth may obviate the need to stay in increasingly over-burdened hospitals with a heightened Covid-19 transmission risk, such a choice may be contraindicated for higher-risk pregnancies, and may go against the wishes of the individual. The lack of clarity heightened these challenges still further; regulations changed rapidly in response to changing transmission rates, rendering it impossible to plan for every contingency. Hospitals also had to make difficult choices around risk management, balancing patient choice with safety, and considering how to deal with symptomatic patients being admitted; how to give them the care that they needed at the lowest risk to others, and in doing so, potentially making it harder to access particular sections of the hospital for those who might have otherwise wanted to use them.

This chapter discusses the impact of the developing pandemic on the stages of maternity, from ante-natal appointments and pregnancy itself, through labour and delivery and the post-partum period. The article will take a socio-cultural and auto-ethnographic approach, taking into account the academic backgrounds of the authors, as well as one author's personal experience of pregnancy and childbirth during the pandemic. The chapter recognises the ongoing nature of the pandemic; we do not claim to offer an exhaustive account or analysis, and we largely restrict ourselves to the UK context.

Pregnancy and Ante-Natal Care

The Covid-19 pandemic had significant impacts upon the provision of antenatal services, and also curtailed the possibilities available as preparations were made for birth. In the UK, patient choice and shared decision-making between patient and clinician constitute a key component of the NHS's long-term plan.[3] However, in many cases, the restrictions imposed by the pandemic limited the choices available to patients. This put families at risk of feeling isolated and disempowered, threatening their experiences of the care received and leading to increased stress and anxiety. In the UK context, hospitals were faced with a set of sometimes conflicting priorities: they needed to conform to government guidelines, while also providing particular standards of care (including offering a degree of patient

---

3 NHS England, 'Shared Decision Making,' https://www.england.nhs.uk/shared-decision-making/, accessed January 12, 2023.

choice), while safeguarding both patients and staff from infection. The relative autonomy given to individual hospitals led them to adjust their advice in ways that had significant impacts on pregnancies. Consultants at Royal Hampshire County Hospital, for example, fluctuated in their advice on whether potential vaginal birth after caesarean (VBAC) candidates should be encouraged to opt for elective caesareans or go forward with a trial of labour after caesarean (TOLAC). As Carauleanu et al. note,[4] the 'paucity of resources' available to hospitals during the pandemic represented a further challenge, as these needed to be balanced with safeguarding 'the fundamental rights and ethical principles' involved in making this decision. This introduced further anxiety for patients who were already faced with such a significant decision.

The risk of contracting Covid-19 during pregnancy represented a further source of anxiety. Symptomatic Covid-19 in pregnancy is correlated with 'higher rates of adverse outcomes, including maternal mortality, preeclampsia, and preterm birth compared with pregnant individuals without COVID-19 diagnosis'; similarly, babies born to Covid-positive patients have a higher risk of severe complications or death.[5] Pregnant people therefore had further cause to be vigilant around Covid-19, and this is likely to have had an impact on their willingness to access care if seeking reassurance. From an infectivity perspective, the safest situation was a complication-free pregnancy, which could limit the amount of time spent in hospital. More than ever, pregnant people were expected to decide for themselves whether a worrisome symptom deserved medical attention.

The measures taken to slow the spread of Covid-19 also had significant effects of the way communication between healthcare professionals, patients and their families was conducted. Even something as simple as the introduction of masks could represent an example of this. Previous research has suggested that face masks may pose challenges for verbal communication and processing,[6] as well as for emotion recognition and comprehension.[7] One study in the Hong Kong context even indicated that a

---

4 Alexandru Carauleanu et al., 'Professional Ethics, VBAC And COVID-19 Pandemic: A Challenge To Be Resolved (Review),' *Experimental and Therapeutic Medicine* 22:3 (2021): 956. https://doi.org/10.3892/etm.2021.10388.

5 José Villar et. al. 'Maternal and Neonatal Morbidity and Mortality Among Pregnant Women With and Without COVID–19 Infection,' *JAMA Pediatrics* 175:8 (2021): 817–826.

6 Mandfred Spitzer, 'Masked Education? The Benefits And Burdens Of Wearing Face Masks In Schools During The Current Corona Pandemic,' *Trends in Neuroscience and Education* 20 (2020): https://doi.org/10.1016%2Fj.tine.2020.100138.

7 Marta Calbi et al., 'The Consequences Of COVID-19 On Social Interactions: An Online Study On Face Covering,' *Scientific Reports* 11:1 (2021): 2601; Claus-Christian Carbon, 'Wearing Face Masks Strongly Confuses Counterparts in Reading Emotions,' *Frontiers in Psychology* 11 (2020), https://doi.org/10.3389%2Ffpsyg.2020.566886; Erez Freud et al, 'The COVID-19 Pandemic Masks The Way

doctor's use of a facemask had a negative effect on patients' perceptions of the doctor's empathy.[8] It is therefore reasonable to assume that face masks, while instrumental in reducing infectivity, may have a negative effect on the rapport between patient and healthcare professional, leading to further anxiety. The modality of communication in some contexts also changed, with telehealth used in both the prenatal and neonatal care contexts, which may have caused further uncertainty.

All these issues were exacerbated by government communications which were at times confusing or contradictory.[9] Public trust in the government's messaging declined as the pandemic progressed, as did trust in the news,[10] leading to further uncertainty and anxiety for care-givers and –receivers alike. The pandemic therefore brought a constellation of anxieties, including but not limited to the fear of infection for both oneself and the baby, anxieties around the availability of desired options for labour, and the risk of curtailed prenatal care, all overlaid by the uncertainty caused by unclear governmental communication and the threat of isolation due to partners being restricted from pre-natal appointments. Of course, pregnant people also faced the same anxieties around Covid-19 as those who were not pregnant, which could range from anxieties over financial security, job security, and the health and wellbeing of oneself and one's loved ones.[11]

It is therefore unsurprising that Covid-19 was shown to have a significant effect on the mental health of pregnant people, evidenced by increased anxiety and depression scores compared to pre-pandemic scores.[12] Research from the Greek context similarly indicated significant increases in the anxiety levels of pregnant people during the pandemic, with the greatest increase being noted in the first

---

People Perceive Faces,' *Scientific Reports* 10:1 (2020): 22344, https://www.nature.com/articles/s41598-020-78986-9; Spitzer, 'Masked Education?'.

8 Carmen Ka Man Wong et al., 'Effect Of Facemasks On Empathy And Relational Continuity: A Randomised Controlled Trial In Primary Care', *BMC Family Practice*, 14:200 (2013), https://doi.org/10.1186/1471-2296-14-200.

9 Stephen Cushion et. al. 'Coronavirus: Fake Less of a Problem Than Confusing Government Messages,' *The Conversation*, 12 June 2020, https://theconversation.com/coronavirus-fake-news-less-of-a-problem-than-confusing-government-messages-new-study-140383, accessed 21 December 2021.

10 Richard Fletcher et. al. 'Information Inequality In The UK Coronavirus Communications Crisis,' *Reuters Institute for the Study of Journalism*, 23 July 2020, https://reutersinstitute.politics.ox.ac.uk/information-inequality-uk-coronavirus-communications-crisis, accessed 13 April 2023.

11 Nader Salari et al. 'Prevalence Of Stress, Anxiety, Depression Among The General Population During The COVID-19 Pandemic: A Systematic Review And Meta-Analysis', *Globalization and Health* 16:1 (2020): 1–11, https://doi.org/10.1186/s12992-020-00589-w.

12 Rasha. E. Khamees, et al. 'Anxiety And Depression During Pregnancy In The Era Of COVID–19,' *Journal of Perinatal Medicine* 49(6) (2021): 674–677, https://doi.org/10.1515/jpm-2021-0181.

week of lockdown.[13] Similar findings were reported in the US context, with participants reporting increased levels of stress, anxiety, and depression.[14]

Pregnancy Loss

Any discussion of the pandemic's effects on pregnancy needs to consider the possibility of pregnancy loss. While it is generally hoped that a pregnancy ends with a positive outcome, pregnancy loss is a very real risk, with the UK National Health Service (NHS) estimating that across the UK, approximately 1 in 6 known pregnancies end in miscarriage, approximately 1 in every 200 births is a stillbirth, and approximately 2000 terminations for reasons of foetal abnormality are performed each year. These figures are available on the NHS website. Of all forms of bereavement, the loss of a wanted pregnancy can bring particular challenges; the loss is usually sudden and unexpected,[15] entailing an intensely embodied experience where the loss is both physical and mental.[16] Enduring societal taboos around the subject lead some bereaved parents to feel isolated in their grief, feeling that conventions, norms and cultural scripts around bereavement are not appropriate to their situation.[17]

The pandemic further exacerbated these challenges.[18] Hospital support was affected by coronavirus restrictions, with many hospitals limiting the number of appointments for scans; if a pregnant person was experiencing symptoms they feared could be a miscarriage, therefore, it was not guaranteed that they would

---

13 Themistoklis Dagklis et al. 'Anxiety During Pregnancy In The Era Of The COVID-19 Pandemic.' *The Lancet* (2020): preprint.

14 Carolyn R. Ahlers-Schmidt et al., 'Concerns Of Women Regarding Pregnancy And Childbirth During The COVID-19 Pandemic,' *Patient Education and Counseling*, 103:12 (2020): 2578–2582, https://doi.org/10.1016%2Fj.pec.2020.09.031.

15 Anette Kersting and Birgit Wagner, 'Complicated Grief After Perinatal Loss,' *Dialogues in Clinical Neuroscience* 14:2 (2012): 187–194.

16 Jeanette Littlemore and Sarah Turner, 'What Can Metaphor Tell Us About Experiences of Pregnancy Loss and How Are These Experiences Reflected in Midwife Practice?' *Frontiers in Communication* 4 (2012): 42.

17 Catherine Hackett Renner et al. 'The Meaning Of Miscarriage To Others: Is It An Unrecognized Loss?' *Journal of Personal & Interpersonal Loss* 5:1 (2000): 65–76; Littlemore and Turner, 'What Can Metaphor Tell Us'.

18 Sergio A. Silverio et al. on behalf of the PUDDLES Global Collaboration, 'Preliminary Findings On The Experiences Of Care For Parents Who Suffered Perinatal Bereavement During The COVID-19 Pandemic,' *BMC Pregnancy and Childbirth* 21:840 (2021) https://doi.org/10.1186/s12884-021-04292-5.

be offered a scan to check. Partners were not always allowed to attend appointments, meaning that bad news was often delivered to the pregnant person alone, without the support of their partner. Hospitals' response to the pandemic had an impact on the care that was offered in the case of a miscarriage; missed or incomplete miscarriages and anembryonic pregnancy were more likely to be offered 'expectant' management, or medical management at home, rather than being treated in hospital.[19] Families experiencing such losses reported that they oscillated between wanting to have control over what was happening, and allowing the situation to progress naturally. Their attitudes in this regard had an impact on the types or levels of support they needed, with some parents appreciating more directive guidance, and others needing to be given a choice.[20] Given the curtailed support offered, it is likely that healthcare staff would find it even harder to provide such individualised care.

The lockdowns resulted in isolation and loneliness for many,[21] conditions that are particularly problematic in the context of grief. Social support has been attested as a key component in managing grief,[22] and while online provision was an appropriate substitute for many, others may have benefited less from this. As the pandemic progressed, it is likely that if a bereaved parent chose to seek support from one of the more general bereavement support charities, as opposed to one specifically dealing with pregnancy loss, they may find themselves needing to contend with long waiting times as the rising death rates led more people to seek the support these services offered.[23] Even if a bereaved parent chose to rely on family and friends for support, the heightened levels of anxiety, stress and depression overall may mean that previously dependable members of a support network were no longer able to provide the level of care expected; 'caregiver fatigue' and burnout, for example, are more likely when a caregiver cannot take adequate time to care for themselves. Research into end-of-life care and bereavement more generally indicated that the pandemic had a demonstrably negative effect on the bereaved's abilities to obtain support from their loved ones. This was due to a

---

19 Miscarriage Association, 'Coronavirus and Miscarriage,' https://www.miscarriageassociation.org.uk/information/information-on-coronavirus-covid-19/, accessed 12 January 2023.

20 Littlemore and Turner, 'What Can Metaphor Tell Us'; Jeannette Littlemore & Sarah Turner, 'Metaphors in communication about pregnancy loss,' *Metaphor and the Social World,* 10:1 (2020): 45–75, https://doi.org/10.1075/msw.18030.lit.

21 Salari et al., 'Prevalence Of Stress.'

22 L. P. Riley, et al. 'Parental Grief Responses And Personal Growth Following The Death Of A Child,' *Death Studies* 31:4 (2007): 277–299.

23 Emily Harrop et al., 'Support Needs And Barriers To Accessing Support: Baseline Results Of A Mixed-Methods National Survey Of People Bereaved During The COVID-19 Pandemic,' *Palliative Medicine* 35:10 (2021): 1985–1997.

range of factors, including the inability to meet together, the heightened stress levels in family members, or the bereaved person's own reticence to ask for help; as one participant explained, 'It has sometimes made it hard to ask for help when I am aware that everyone is having a difficult time due to COVID'.[24]

Finally, funeral and memorialisation options following a loss were also curtailed. For some bereaved through pregnancy loss, having a funeral or memorialisation service is particularly important, as it provides a means of affirming the deceased baby as having had a unique identity – even if the loss occurred at a relatively early gestational age.[25] The restrictions imposed on funerary provisions meant that these opportunities were no longer available.

The pandemic, therefore, is likely to have made the experience of pregnancy loss even more difficult. It is possible that these compounding factors may also increase the risk of complex grief, which is exacerbated by losses in traumatic situations and where support following the loss is inadequate.[26] Pregnancy loss is already often highly traumatic, but the pandemic's negative effects on support provision are likely to put those who suffer such a loss at increased risk.

Labour and Delivery

The pregnancy and childbirth journey is a fluctuating admixture of medical care and otherwise natural processes, throughout which medical invention may be necessary at any time. However, the pandemic further complicated the relationship between the medical and the 'natural', impacting upon how an individual's decisions around their care may lean more towards one or the other. For example, a person who formerly put faith in the safety of the medical environment might now feel that such a choice was the riskiest due to the risk of Covid-19 infection; likewise, a patient who had hoped for a home birth may have found that it would no longer be possible because of the risks, and incompatibility with restrictions, for all involved. More generally, the pandemic brought challenges to the practical arrangements required throughout pregnancy and during labour. Expectant parents were, like the rest of the population, advised to avoid public transport; those without personal cars may therefore have felt that they were putting their unborn child (and themselves) at risk. Those with existing children worried about where to send them at the onset of labour; situations arose where

---

24 Harrop et al. 'Support Needs.'

25 Littlemore and Turner, 'What Can Metaphor Tell Us.'

26 Kersting and Wagner, 'Complicated Grief.'

families had to choose which family or friends to put at risk, those without them were given no clear advice on what to do. Partners risked missing births while sitting outside in the carpark with siblings-to-be.

Thus, the measures put in place to slow the spread of Covid-19 brought with them a number of ethical challenges related to labour and delivery arrangements. The need to protect healthcare workers, patients, and newborn babies from Covid-19 needed to be balanced with the need for pregnant people and their partners to be supported through the physical and emotional challenges of childbirth.[27] Research into post-partum PTSD, a condition affecting 3–4% of pregnancies,[28] has identified three risk factors which seem particular relevant to a discussion of the impact of Covid-19 on childbirth: a perceived lack of control during the birth, a lack of support from partner and/or medical staff, and a negative gap between the expectation and the reality of the birth process.[29] The limitations imposed by the Covid-19 restrictions are likely to have exacerbated each of these risk factors, with patients curtailed in their options for labour and delivery and/or denied the presence of a birth partner, leading to their actual experience of the birth being very different to what they may have hoped for. The possibility of developing PTSD is particularly problematic given that the context is not one that is normally associated with trauma, but rather with positive outlooks; a new parent has the pressure to conform to ideas and ideals of the arrival of a child, which can entail judgment for anything less than joy. Going through childbirth can be stressful under any circumstances, but is inherently more traumatic during an emergency situation (including a pandemic). The risk of PTSD is further exacerbated by sleep-deprivation – already common in the early days of parenthood, and worsened by the pandemic for some.[30] The isolation of lockdown heightened the risk still further.

To give an example of the ways in which the pandemic negatively impacted choices offered around labour and delivery, some UK hospitals responded to the pandemic by restricting the provision of elective caesareans.[31] This posed problems, as many elective caesareans, while not clinically 'necessary', are requested due to health

---

27 Nofar Yakovi Gan-Or, 'Going Solo: The Law And Ethics Of Childbirth During The COVID–19 Pandemic,' *Journal of Law and the Biosciences* 7:1 (2020): 1–17.

28 Antje Horsch and Susan Garthus-Niegel, 'Posttraumatic Stress Disorder Following Childbirth,' in *Childbirth, Vulnerability and Law: Exploring Issues of Violence and Control*, ed. Camilla Pickles and Jonathan Herring (London: Routledge, 2019).

29 Horsch and Garthus-Niegel, 'Posttraumatic Stress.'

30 Horsch and Garthus–Niegel, 'Posttraumatic Stress.'; Andy J. King, et. al. 'The Challenge Of Maintaining Metabolic Health During A Global Pandemic,' *Sports Medicine* 50 (2020): 1233–1241, https://doi.org/10.1007/s40279-020-01295-8.

31 Note that the cap on c-sections has now been removed as it was a cause of harm. See BMJ 2022: https://www.bmj.com/content/376/bmj.o446, accessed 13 April 2023.

conditions which could be worsened by vaginal delivery, or due to previous traumatic experiences such as sexual assault or previous negative birth experiences.[32]
Removing this choice further jeopardised the birthing experience, putting the pregnant person at risk of further trauma and post-partum mental health issues. At one
point, too, requests for elective caesareans seemed to be on the rise as a mitigation to
the rule that partners may only be present during active labour.[33] Similarly, many
homebirthing services were suspended during the pandemic, with one third of NHS
trusts shutting down this provision in March 2020; again, the decreased choice this
entailed is likely to have caused distress, especially given that the need to attend
hospital may lead to heightened anxiety regarding Covid-19 infection. Such a decision may also have led some pregnant people to choose to freebirth (i.e., give birth
without midwifery or medical support) in order to fulfil their wish of giving birth
at home.[34]

In threatening non-birthing partners' ability to be present throughout labour
and birth, the pandemic may also impact upon the creation of family identities. As
Einion-Waller & Regan note, 'childbirth is not just the birth of a baby; it is also the
birth of a family',[35] and the presence of a supportive partner throughout labour
and delivery has been shown to facilitate this process. For example, fathers' participation and presence in labour and birth was considered 'a unique and exclusive
opportunity to bond with their new-born'[36] with important roles also identified in
supporting the pregnant person and advocating for their needs, which in turn in-
duced feelings of involvement and security in fathers.[37] Studies have indicated that
being present at the birth of their child represented a transition to fatherhood[38]

---

32 Elizabeth Chloe Romanis and Anna Nelson, 'Maternal Request Caesareans And COVID-19: The
Virus Does Not Diminish The Importance Of Choice In Childbirth,' *Journal of Medical Ethics* 46:11
(2020): 726–731.
33 Carys Betteley, 'Covid: Pregnant Women "Opt For C-Section" To Ensure Partners At Birth,' *BBC
News*, 26 September 2020, https://www.bbc.co.uk/news/uk-wales-54263166, accessed 15 December 2021.
34 Elizabeth Chloe Romanis and Anna Nelson, 'Homebirthing In The United Kingdom During
COVID-19', *Medical Law International* 20:3 (2020): 183–200, https://doi.org/10.1177/0968533220955224.
35 Alys Einion-Waller and Maeve Regan, '"Knowing That I Had a Choice Empowered Me": Preparing for and Experiencing Birth during a Pandemic,' in *Mothers, Mothering, and COVID-19: Dispatches from the Pandemic*, ed. Fiona Green and Andrea O'Reilly, (Ontario: Demeter Press, 2021).
36 Margareta Johansson, Jennifer Fenwick & Åsa Premberg, 'A Meta–Synthesis Of Fathers' Experiences Of Their Partner's Labour And The Birth Of Their Baby,' *Midwifery* 31:1 (2015): 13.
37 Johansson, Fenwick, and Premberg, 'Fathers' Experiences.'
38 Martin P. Johnson, 'An Exploration Of Men's Experience And Role At Childbirth', *The Journal
of Men's Studies*, 10:2 (2002): 165–182; Heather L. Longworth and Carol K. Kingdon, 'Fathers In
The Birth Room: What Are They Expecting And Experiencing? A Phenomenological Study,' *Midwifery* 27:5 (2011): 588–594.

and a closer familial connection.[39] The father's presence at the birth has also been associated with reductions in pain and anxiety levels, and even shorter labour in some cases,[40] and the presence of a supportive birth partner may also help to ensure that the labouring person's rights to medical autonomy and informed consent are not violated.[41] While this research was specific to fathers, it is reasonable to suggest that such findings could hold true for non-birthing partners of any gender. The negative impacts of the pandemic's restrictions therefore extend beyond the pregnant individual to include partners and, as we will see next, the wider family context.

Post-Partum Period

The post-partum period is an exhausting and at times challenging one, even under normal circumstances. In some cases, these challenges can lead to clinical mental health conditions; post-natal depression, for example, is a known risk following pregnancy, affecting more than one in ten patients within a year of giving birth.[42] It is reasonable to assume that the high levels of disruption and uncertainty engendered by the pandemic may have further heightened the risk of experiencing postnatal depression or anxiety. Indeed, research conducted on postnatal women in the UK indicated high levels of self-reported negative psychosocial changes as a result of social distancing measures, with high rates of 'clinically relevant' maternal depression and anxiety compared to pre-pandemic rates.[43] For some participants in a

---

39 Kerstin Erlandsson and Helena Lindgren, 'From Belonging To Belonging Through A Blessed Moment Of Love For A Child–The Birth Of A Child From The Fathers' Perspective,' *Journal of Men's Health* 6:4 (2009): 338–344.

40 Lars Plantin, Adepeju Olykoya and Pernilla Ny, 'Positive Health Outcomes Of Fathers' Involvement In Pregnancy And Childbirth Paternal Support: A Scope Study Literature Review,' *Fathering: A Journal of Theory, Research, and Practice about Men as Fathers* 9:1 (2011): 87–102.

41 Gan-Or, 'Going Solo.'

42 NHS England, 'Overview – Postnatal Depression,' https://www.nhs.uk/mental-health/conditions/post-natal-depression/overview/, accessed January 12, 2023.

43 Margie Davenport et al. 'Moms Are Not OK: COVID-19 and Maternal Mental Health,' *Frontiers in Global Women's Health*, 1:1 (2020), https://doi.org/10.3389/fgwh.2020.00001; Victoria Fallon et al. 'Psychosocial Experiences Of Postnatal Women During The COVID-19 Pandemic. A UK-Wide Study Of Prevalence Rates And Risk Factors For Clinically Relevant Depression And Anxiety,' *Journal of Psychiatric Research* 136 (2021): 157–166, https://doi.org/10.1016/j.jpsychires.2021.01.048.

study conducted in the US context, depressive symptoms were correlated with lower self-reported levels of bonding with the baby.[44]

There are likely to be a multitude of reasons for these negative impacts upon mental health, ranging from those specific to the pregnancy to those related more broadly to the experience of having lived through such a momentous event as the pandemic. As mentioned above, negative mental health outcomes may be a result of a gap between expectation and reality; while this was introduced in the context of labour and delivery specifically, in many cases, the pandemic had a significant impact on the post-partum period too, leading to a similar 'gap' between expectation and reality. For example, travel restrictions meant that extended family could not meet the new arrivals except over video communication software such as Zoom, and as the pandemic wore on, culturally significant milestones were missed or celebrated in a very different way. A family celebrating the first Christmas of their baby born in 2020, for instance, would likely have had to mark the occasion without the presence of extended family as they might have wished.

Not only did the lockdown measures have negative effects on the post-partum period in terms of family bonding, but post-natal care was also impacted. Midwives and health visitors could no longer visit people in their houses, and entering hospitals with a newborn carried a risk of infection. Responsibility for infant and maternal wellbeing fell upon the shoulders of new parents, heightening anxiety[45] The parents became responsible for determining when a worrisome symptom was 'wrong' enough to warrant medical attention;[46] for example, newborn weight checks normally carried out by health visitors were cancelled, unless the parents thought the baby was not gaining weight at a healthy pace, in which case a doorstep weigh-in could be arranged. Furthermore, the health and wellbeing of the healthcare workers themselves had to be taken into account,[47] and every call out added to their strain and risk. Postnatal checks, including those intended to screen for post-partum depression, were moved to Zoom. Breastfeeding support was also negatively affected by Covid-19. While some new parents appreciated the increased time at home (and fewer visitors), others struggled to get support when the experienced challenges

---

44 Cindy H. Liu et al. 'Psychological Risks To Mother–Infant Bonding During The COVID-19 Pandemic,' *Pediatric Research* 91 (2022): 853–861, https://doi.org/10.1038/s41390-021-01751-9.
45 Karleen Gribble et al. 'Implications of the COVID-19 Pandemic Response for Breastfeeding, Maternal Caregiving Capacity and Infant Mental Health', *Journal of Human Lactation,* 36(4) (2020), https://doi.org/10.1177/0890334420949514.
46 Silverio, Jackson et al. 'Psychological Experiences.'
47 Alyce N. Wilson et al. 'Caring For The Carers: Ensuring The Provision Of Quality Maternity Care During A Global Pandemic,' *Women and Birth* 34:3 (2021): 206–209, https://doi.org/10.1016%2Fj.wombi.2020.03.011.

with breastfeeding, leading some to stop breastfeeding before they were ready.[48] Parents of babies requiring neonatal intensive care were strongly affected, as in some cases the time they were permitted to spend visiting their baby was limited, affecting the establishment of a milk supply.[49]

The pandemic did not only bring disadvantages to post-partum life, however. In many cases, partners, who would normally have been expected to return to work after their period of leave, could now be physically present with their new family. While baby groups are a source of support and comfort to some, for others they are an unwanted source of social pressure that was relieved through the confinement of lockdown. Where new parents might have felt obliged to host family to meet their new arrival, they now had the opportunity to impose privacy in the early days, allowing themselves to enjoy their baby alone. For most people it was likely a mixed experience. Public and academic responses showed this admixture of relief and isolation; for example, James Kent's 2021 *Pregnant during a Pandemic* project photographed parents and families' responses to lockdown and beyond. A participant in this project ambiguously expressed that she felt she had 'given birth to a secret baby, behind closed doors'.[50] This aspect of being 'hidden' or 'secret' could be a burden, a blessing, or both. Similarly, a participant in Kristopher Lovell's *#RecordCovid19* project described her early post-partum period in an admixture of emotions:

> March 30th, I'm sat stunned in my living room with a premature baby who came home after 3.5 months in hospital only to be straight into lockdown with him. We're shielded because he's on oxygen with COPD and I am genuinely frozen in shock because I don't know how to process what this means for everyday life. [. . .] My neighbours communicate from the window, they tap and I instantly hold the baby up to the window. They mouth 'do I need anything' and I always say 'I'm fine'. This is my routine. But oddly it's a lovely one. And I'm 100% sure the baby is their ray of light too. Before covid how many neighbours did this. Like everyone else, I hope the community spirit prevails. Though the antisocial part of me hopes a 2m distance is a permanent feature. At this point, I've no idea how I'll ever return to 'normal'.[51]

---

48 Amy Brown & Natalie Shenker, 'Experiences Of Breastfeeding During COVID-19: Lessons For Future Practical And Emotional Support,' *Maternal & Child Nutrition*, 17:1 (2021): e13088, https://doi.org/10.1111/mcn.13088.

49 Cecília Tomori et al. 'When Separation Is Not The Answer: Breastfeeding Mothers And Infants Affected By COVID-19,' *Maternal & Child Nutrition*, 16:4 (2020): e13033, https://doi.org/10.1111/mcn.13033.

50 James Clifford Kent and Sarah Lloyd-Fox, 'Generation COVID: Pregnancy, Birth And Postnatal Life In The Pandemic,' *The Conversation*, 15 July 2021, https://theconversation.com/generation-covid-pregnancy-birth-and-postnatal-life-in-the-pandemic-160644, accessed 10 December 2021.

51 [*#RecordCovid19*-85] Cambridgeshire, Content Writer, Female, 35, http://kristopherlovell.com/2020/10/05/recordcovid19-85-cambridgeshire-content-writer-female-35/, accessed 13 April 2023.

For this participant, the shock of lockdown, combined with the pressures of caring for a vulnerable baby, is juxtaposed with what she considers positive developments in 'community spirit'. Despite these positive aspects, however, the uncertainty remains; a return to 'normal' seems impossible for her. While the journey to parenthood always entails significant upheaval, there is no doubt that the pandemic brought further challenges.

Conclusion

The coronavirus pandemic has had, undeniably, a significant impact on society as a whole. However, we have argued here that the challenges brought about by the pandemic had particular consequences for pregnant people and their families. Lockdown restrictions curtailed the choices available, and put pregnant people at risk of isolation at all stages of the pregnancy journey. Desired options for labour could not always be accommodated, and uncertainty around the available options and the risk factors entailed by each led to anxiety. The support available in both pre – and post-natal contexts was changed or limited, with face-to-face provision becoming harder to come by. The social lives of new parents were impacted by lockdown restrictions, and it became harder to draw on support networks in the face of challenges. All these challenges were exacerbated by unclear communication, leading to further ambiguity.

In the UK context, too, the actions of the government led to anger as these seemed contradictory to the regulations which had been put in place. In May 2020, Dominic Cummings, then chief adviser to PM Boris Johnson, was criticised for breaking lockdown restrictions and driving his family to his parents' farm in County Durham while experiencing Covid-19 symptoms. Boris Johnson defended him as having acted 'legally, responsibly and with integrity'; 'any father, any parent', he claimed, would understand what he did'.[52] A participant in Lovell's *#RecordCovid19* project wrote to their MP expressing their exasperation with the situation, writing that:

> Mr Johnson's ludicrous defence of Cummings as having acted with 'integrity' to follow his 'fatherly instinct' is, to put it colloquially, a slap in the face to all parents who have reluctantly put their 'parental instincts' aside and chosen to follow the lockdown regulations instead. Many parents have been forced to care for their children while they themselves are

---

52 Jedidajah Otte and Aaron Walawalkar, 'UK Coronavirus Live: Boris Johnson Says Dominic Cummings Acted "Responsibly, Legally And With Integrity" – As It Happened,' *The Guardian*, 24 May 2020, https://www.theguardian.com/world/live/2020/may/24/uk-coronavirus-live-dominic-cummings-under-intense-pressure-over-lockdown-breaches, accessed 12 January 2023.

sick; been unable to see their children when they themselves are symptomatic; and in some cases been unable to visit their sick and dying children [. . .]

Mr Johnson has effectively, in mounting this defence of Cummings, criticised all those parents who have been forced to make unfathomable decisions regarding their own children in order to protect the safety and lives of their fellow citizens. This, once more, is simply unconscionable; a nation already in mourning for so many of its loved ones does not deserve to, in effect, be told that they failed their children by doing what they were previously told was the only right and correct thing to do.[53]

The elements that this participant highlights mirror the issues found in the discussion of the ante-, peri – and post-natal stages; parents of children of any age were forced to make difficult decisions between restricted options, with little clear communication to guide them, even in the face of clear disregard for regulations by members of the government. Interestingly, there was a complete lack of clarity about the legitimacy of 'breaking' restrictions for reasons of childcare support, something that only became widely advertised once Johnson had welcomed his own pandemic baby.

Looking to the future, the long-term ramifications of the pandemic remain to be seen. However, those who were pregnant during the pandemic, and their families, are likely to feel the effects of the increased levels of anxiety and depression for some time to come. Research has already indicated that the pandemic may have effects on the development of babies too,[54] pointing to long-term implications for the next generation as well as the current. While pessimism is not warranted, it is undeniable that we will be living with Covid-19 and the effects of its arrival for years to come. Perhaps it is apposite here to echo the words of the participant above: 'At this point, I have no idea how I'll ever return to "normal"'. We can, however, use the lessons learned from this pandemic to work towards better maternal and neonatal care, and to support more effectively those affected by the upheavals of Covid-19.

---

53 [*#RecordCovid19*-57] Wales, Writer, Female, 28, http://kristopherlovell.com/2020/05/26/recordcovid19-57-wales-writer-female-28/, accessed 13 April 2023.

54 Lauren C. Shuffrey et al. 'Association Of Birth During The COVID-19 Pandemic With Neurodevelopmental Status At 6 Months In Infants With And Without In Utero Exposure To Maternal SARS-Cov-2 Infection,' *JAMA Pediatrics* 176:6 (2022): e215563–e215563.

References

Ahlers-Schmidt, Carolyn R., Ashley M. Hervey, Tara Neil, Stephanie Kuhlmann, and Zachary Kuhlmannd. 'Concerns Of Women Regarding Pregnancy And Childbirth During The COVID-19 Pandemic.' *Patient Education and Counseling* 103:12 (2020): 2578–2582. https://doi.org/10.1016%2Fj.pec.2020.09.031

Alehagen, Siw., Barbro Wijma, Ulf Lundberg, Klaas Wijma. 'Fear, Pain And Stress Hormones During Childbirth.' *Journal of Psychosomatic Obstetrics & Gynecology*, 26:3 (2005): 153–165. https://doi.org/10.1080/01443610400023072

Betteley, Carys. 'Covid: Pregnant Women "Opt For C-Section" To Ensure Partners At Birth.' *BBC News*, 26 September 2020. https://www.bbc.co.uk/news/uk-wales-54263166. Accessed 15 December 2021.

Brown, Amy and Natalie Shenker. 'Experiences Of Breastfeeding During COVID-19: Lessons For Future Practical And Emotional Support.' *Maternal & Child Nutrition* 17:1 (2021): e13088, https://doi.org/10.1111/mcn.13088.

Calbi, Marta., Nunzio Langiulli, Francesca Ferroni, Martina Montalti, Anna Kolesnikov, Vittorio Gallese & Maria Alessandra Umiltà. 'The Consequences Of COVID-19 On Social Interactions: An Online Study On Face Covering.' *Scientific Reports*, 11:1 (2021): 2601. https://doi.org/10.1038/s41598-021-81780-w.

Carbon, Claus-Christian. 'Wearing Face Masks Strongly Confuses Counterparts in Reading Emotions.' *Frontiers in Psychology* 11 (2020) https://doi.org/10.3389%2Ffpsyg.2020.566886.

Carauleanu, Alexandru., Ingrid Andrada Tanasa, Dragos Nemescu, and Demetra Socolov. 'Professional Ethics, VBAC And COVID-19 Pandemic: A Challenge To Be Resolved (Review).' *Experimental and Therapeutic Medicine* 22:3 (2021): 956.

Cushion, Stephen., Maria Kyriakidou, Marina Morani and Nikki Soo. 'Coronavirus: Fake News Less of a Problem Than Confusing Government Messages.' *The Conversation*, 12 June 2020. https://theconversation.com/coronavirus-fake-news-less-of-a-problem-than-confusing-government-messages-new-study-140383. Accessed 21 December 2021.

Dagklis, Themistoklis., Ioannis Tsakiridis, Apostolos Mamopoulos, Apostolos Athanasiadis and Georgios Papazisis. 'Anxiety During Pregnancy In The Era Of The COVID-19 Pandemic.' *The Lancet* (2020): preprint. Available at SSRN: https://ssrn.com/abstract=3588542.

Davenport, Margie. H., Sarah Meyer, Victoria L. Meah, Morgan C. Strynadka and Rshmi Khurana, 'Moms Are Not OK: COVID-19 and Maternal Mental Health.' *Frontiers in Global Women's Health* 1 (2020): 1. https://doi.org/10.3389/fgwh.2020.00001.

Einion-Waller, Alys and Maeve Regan. '"Knowing That I Had a Choice Empowered Me": Preparing for and Experiencing Birth during a Pandemic.' *Mothers, Mothering, and COVID-19: Dispatches from the Pandemic*, edited by Fiona Green and Andrea O'Reilly Ontario: Demeter Press, 2021.

Erlandsson, Kerstin and Helena Lindgren. 'From Belonging To Belonging Through A Blessed Moment Of Love For A Child–The Birth Of A Child From The Fathers' Perspective.' *Journal of Men's Health* 6(4) (2009): 338–344.

Fallon, Victoria., Siân M. Davies, Sergio A. Silverio, Leanne Jackson, Leonardo De Pascalis and Joanne A. Harrold. 'Psychosocial Experiences Of Postnatal Women During The COVID-19 Pandemic. A UK-Wide Study Of Prevalence Rates And Risk Factors For Clinically Relevant Depression And Anxiety.' *Journal of Psychiatric Research* 136 (2021): 157–166. https://doi.org/10.1016/j.jpsychires.2021.01.048.

Fletcher, Richard., Antonis Kalogeropoulos, Felix Simon, and Rasmus Kleis Nielsen. 'Information Inequality In The UK Coronavirus Communications Crisis.' *Reuters Institute for the Study of Journalism*, 23 July 2020. https://reutersinstitute.politics.ox.ac.uk/information-inequality-uk-coronavirus-communications-crisis. Accessed 13 April 2023.

Freud, Erez., Andreja Stajduhar, R. Shayna Rosenbaum, Galia Avidan and Tzvi Ganel. 'The COVID-19 Pandemic Masks The Way People Perceive Faces.' *Scientific Reports* 10:1 (2020): 22344. https://doi.org/10.1038/s41598-020-78986-9.

Gan-Or, Nofar Yakovi. 'Going Solo: The Law And Ethics Of Childbirth During The COVID-19 Pandemic.' *Journal of Law and the Biosciences* 9:1 (2020): 1–17. https://doi.org/10.1093/jlb/lsaa079.

General Medical Council. 'Decision Making and Consent.' https://www.gmc-uk.org/ethical-guidance/ethical-guidance-for-doctors/decision-making-and-consent. Accessed 12 January 2023.

Gribble, Karleen., Kathleen A. Marinelli, Cecília Tomori and Marielle S. Gross, 'Implications of the COVID-19 Pandemic Response for Breastfeeding, Maternal Caregiving Capacity and Infant Mental Health.' *Journal of Human Lactation* 36:4 (2020).https://doi.org/10.1177/0890334420949514.

Otte, Jedidajah and Aaron Walawalkar, 'UK Coronavirus Live: Boris Johnson Says Dominic Cummings Acted "Responsibly, Legally And With Integrity" – As It Happened.' *The Guardian*, 24 May 2020. https://www.theguardian.com/world/live/2020/may/24/uk-coronavirus-live-dominic-cummings-under-intense-pressure-over-lockdown-breaches. Accessed 12 January 2023.

Harrop, Emily., Silvia Goss, Damian Farnell, Mirella Longo, Anthony Byrne, Kali Barawi, Anna Torrens-Burton, Annmarie Nelson, Kathy Seddon, Linda Machin, Eileen Sutton, Audrey Roulston, Anne Finucane, Alison Penny, Kirsten V Smith, Stephanie Sivell and Lucy E Selman. 'Support Needs And Barriers To Accessing Support: Baseline Results Of A Mixed-Methods National Survey Of People Bereaved During The COVID-19 Pandemic.' *Palliative Medicine* 35:10 (2021): 1985–1997. https://doi.org/10.1177/02692163211043372.

Horsch, Antje and Susan Garthus-Niegel. 'Posttraumatic Stress Disorder Following Childbirth.' In *Childbirth, Vulnerability and Law: Exploring Issues of Violence and Control*, edited by Camilla Pickles and Jonathan Herring. London: Routledge, 2019.

Johansson, Margareta., Jennifer Fenwick and Åsa Premberg. 'A Meta-Synthesis Of Fathers' Experiences Of Their Partner'S Labour And The Birth Of Their Baby.' *Midwifery* 31:1 (2015): 9–18.

Johnson, Martin P. 'An Exploration Of Men's Experience And Role At Childbirth.' *The Journal of Men's Studies*, 10:2 (2002): 165–182.

Kent, James Clifford. *Pregnant in a Pandemic* (2021). https://www.jckent.com/pregnant-in-a-pandemic/. Accessed 10 December 2021.

Kent, James Clifford and Sarah Lloyd-Fox. 'Generation COVID: Pregnancy, Birth And Postnatal Life In The Pandemic.' *The Conversation*, 15 July 2021, https://theconversation.com/generation-covid-pregnancy-birth-and-postnatal-life-in-the-pandemic-160644. Accessed 10 December 2021.

Kersting, Anette and Birgit Wagner. 'Complicated Grief After Perinatal Loss.' *Dialogues in Clinical Neuroscience* 14:2 (2012): 187–194.

Khamees, Rasha. E., Omima Taha and Tamer Yehia M. Ali 'Anxiety And Depression During Pregnancy In The Era Of COVID-19.' *Journal of Perinatal Medicine* 49:6 (2021): 674–677. https://doi.org/10.1515/jpm-2021-0181.

King, Andy. J., Louise M. Burke, Shona L. Halson and John A. Hawley. 'The Challenge Of Maintaining Metabolic Health During A Global Pandemic.' *Sports Medicine* 50 (2020): 1233–1241. https://doi.org/10.1007/s40279-020-01295-8.

Littlemore, Jeanette and Sarah Turner. 'What Can Metaphor Tell Us About Experiences of Pregnancy Loss and How Are These Experiences Reflected in Midwife Practice?' *Frontiers in Communication* 4 (2019) 42.

Littlemore, Jeanette and Sarah Turner. 'Metaphors In Communication About Pregnancy Loss.' *Metaphor and the Social World* 10:1 (2020): 45–75. https://doi.org/10.1075/msw.18030.lit.

Liu, Cindy H., Sunah Hyun, Leena Mittal and Carmina Erdei, 'Psychological Risks To Mother–Infant Bonding During The COVID-19 Pandemic.' *Pediatric Research* 91 (2021): 853–861.https://doi.org/10.1038/s41390-021-01751-9

Longworth, Heather L and Carol K Kingdon. 'Fathers In The Birth Room: What Are They Expecting And Experiencing? A Phenomenological Study.' *Midwifery* 27:5 (2011): 588–594.

Miscarriage Association. 'Coronavirus and Miscarriage.' https://www.miscarriageassociation.org.uk/information/information-on-coronavirus-covid-19/. Accessed January 12, 2023.

NHS England. 'Shared Decision Making.' https://www.england.nhs.uk/shared-decision-making/. Accessed 12 January 2023.

NHS England. 'Miscarriage.' www.nhs.uk/conditions/Miscarriage/Pages/Introduction.aspx. Accessed 12 January 2023.

NHS England. 'Overview – Postnatal Depression.' https://www.nhs.uk/mental-health/conditions/post-natal-depression/overview/. Accessed 12 January 2023.

Plantin, Lars., Olykoya, Adepeju and Pernilla Ny. 'Positive Health Outcomes Of Fathers' Involvement In Pregnancy And Childbirth Paternal Support: A Scope Study Literature Review.' *Fathering: A Journal of Theory, Research, and Practice about Men as Fathers* 9:1 (2011): 87–102.

Renner, Catherine Hackett., Sophia Verdekal, Sigal Brier and Gina Fallucca. 'The Meaning Of Miscarriage To Others: Is It An Unrecognized Loss?' *Journal of Personal & Interpersonal Loss* 5:1 (2000): 65–76.

Riley, Linda P., Lynda L. LaMontagne, Joseph T. Hepworth and Barbara A. Murphy. 'Parental Grief Responses And Personal Growth Following The Death Of A Child.' *Death Studies* 31:4 (2007): 277–299.

Romanis, Elizabeth Chloe and Anna Nelson. 'Maternal Request Caesareans And COVID-19: The Virus Does Not Diminish The Importance Of Choice In Childbirth.' *Journal of Medical Ethics* 46:11 (2020): 726–731.

Romanis, Elizabeth Chloe and Anna Nelson. 'Homebirthing In The United Kingdom During COVID-19.' *Medical Law International* 20:3 (2020): 183–200.

Salari, Nader., Amin Hosseinian-Far, Rostam Jalali, Aliakbar Vaisi-Raygani, Shna Rasoulpoor, Masoud Mohammadi, Shabnam Rasoulpoor and Behnam Khaledi-Paveh. 'Prevalence Of Stress, Anxiety, Depression Among The General Population During The COVID-19 Pandemic: A Systematic Review And Meta-Analysis.' *Globalization and Health* 16:1 (2020): 1–11.

Shuffrey, Lauren C., Morgan R. Firestein, Margaret H. Kyle, Andrea Fields, Carmela Alcántara, Dima Amso, Judy Austin, Jennifer M. Bain, Jennifer Barbosa, Mary Bence, Catherine Bianco, Cristina R. Fernández, Sylvie Goldman, Cynthia Gyamfi-Bannerman, Violet Hott, Yunzhe Hu, Maha Hussain, Pam Factor-Litvak, Maristella Lucchini, Arthur Mandel, Rachel Marsh, Danielle McBrian, Mirella Mourad, Rebecca Muhle, Kimberly G. Noble, Anna A. Penn, Cynthia Rodriguez, Ayesha Sania, Wendy G. Silver, Kally C. O'Reilly, Melissa Stockwell, Nim Tottenham, Martha G. Welch, Noelia Zork, William P. Fifer, Catherine Monk and Dani Dumitriu. 'Association Of Birth During The COVID-19 Pandemic With Neurodevelopmental Status At 6 Months In Infants With And Without In Utero Exposure To Maternal SARS-Cov-2 Infection.' *JAMA Pediatrics* 176: 6 (2022): e215563.

Silverio, Sergio., Abigail Easter, Claire Storey, Davor Jurković and Jane Sandall on behalf of the PUDDLES Global Collaboration. 'Preliminary Findings On The Experiences Of Care For Parents Who Suffered Perinatal Bereavement During The COVID-19 Pandemic.' *BMC Pregnancy and Childbirth* 21:1 (2021): 840. https://doi.org/10.1186/s12884-021-04292-5.

Spitzer, Manfred. 'Masked Education? The Benefits And Burdens Of Wearing Face Masks In Schools During The Current Corona Pandemic.' *Trends in Neuroscience and Education* 20 (2020): 100138. https://doi.org/10.1016/j.tine.2020.100138.

Tomori, Cecília., Karleen Gribble, Aunchalee E.L. Palmquist, Mija-Tesse Ververs and Marielle S. Gross 'When Separation Is Not The Answer: Breastfeeding Mothers And Infants Affected By COVID-19.' *Maternal & Child Nutrition* 16:4 (2020): e13033. https://doi.org/10.1111/mcn.13033.

Villar, José., Shabina Ariff, Robert B. Gunier, Ramachandran Thiruvengadam, Stephen Rauch, Alexey Kholin, Paola Roggero, Federico Prefumo, Marynéa Silva do Vale, Jorge Arturo Cardona-Perez, Nerea Maiz, Irene Cetin, Valeria Savasi, Philippe Deruelle, Sarah Rae Easter, Joanna Sichitiu, Constanza P. Soto Conti, Ernawati Ernawati, Mohak Mhatre, Jagjit Singh Teji, Becky Liu, Carola Capelli, Manuela Oberto, Laura Salazar, Michael G. Gravett, Paolo Ivo Cavoretto, Vincent Bizor Nachinab, Hadiza Galadanci, Daniel Oros, Adejumoke Idowu Ayede, Loïc Sentilhes, Babagana Bako, Mónica Savorani, Hellas Cena, Perla K. García-May, Saturday Etuk, Roberto Casale, Sherief Abd-Elsalam, Satoru Ikenoue, Muhammad Baffah Aminu, Carmen Vecciarelli, Eduardo A. Duro, Mustapha Ado Usman, Yetunde John-Akinola, Ricardo Nieto, Enrico Ferrazzi, Zulfiqar A. Bhutta, Ana Langer, Stephen H. Kennedy and Aris T. Papageorghiou. 'Maternal and Neonatal Morbidity and Mortality Among Pregnant Women With and Without COVID-19 Infection.' *JAMA Pediatrics* 175:8 (2021): 817–826. https://doi.org/10/1001/jamapediatrics.2021.1050.

Wilson, Alyce. N., Claudia Ravaldi, Michelle J.L. Scoullar, Joshua P. Vogel, Rebecca A. Szabo, Jane R.W. Fisher, and Caroline S.E. Homer. 'Caring For The Carers: Ensuring The Provision Of Quality Maternity Care During A Global Pandemic.' *Women and Birth* 34:3 (2021): 206–209. https://doi.org/10.1016/j.wombi.2020.03.011.

Wong, Carmen Ka Man., Benjamin Hon Kei Yip, Stewart Mercer, Sian Griffiths, Kenny Kung, Martin Chi-sang Wong, Josette Chor and Samuel Yeung-shan Wong. 'Effect Of Facemasks On Empathy And Relational Continuity: A Randomised Controlled Trial In Primary Care.' *BMC Family Practice* 14:1 (2013): 200. https://doi.org/10.1186/1471-2296-14-200.

Iro Filippaki and Alexandra Palli

Chapter Four
Narratives of Resilience During the Covid-19 Pandemic: An Interdisciplinary Approach

Introduction

In one of her most famous essays, Virginia Woolf lamented the absence of literary material on the experience of illness. Titled "On being Ill" (1925), Woolf's essay shows the experience of illness as a short circuit to human emotion, romance, and the sublime: I am ill, one says,

> but what does that convey of the great experience; how the world has changed its shape; the tools of business grown remote; the sounds of festival become romantic like a merry-go–round heard across far fields; and friends have changed, some putting on a strange beauty, others deformed to the squatness of toads, while the whole landscape of life lies remote and fair, like the shore seen from a ship far out at sea[1] (Woolf 1925, 34–35).

Woolf uniquely suggested that we resort to poetry to make sense of our experience of illness, but what also stands out in her essay is the special relationship between feeling ill and feeling everything else, as well as the narrativization of those feelings. Since Woolf's time of writing, many literary authors have taken it upon themselves to record the emotions that illnesses trigger,[2] and academic publications, especially after the first year of the Covid-19 pandemic focused on the importance of the public's emotional responses to both existing and impending illness. As has long been established, not only are emotions central to human survival and adaptation, but their study is also essential for understanding the psychological structure of illness itself.[3] A 2022 publication on the relationship between emotion and disease by Rob Boddice and Bettina Hitzer views the emotional experience of illness

---

1 Virginia Woolf. *On Being Ill.* (The Hogarth Press. 1930 [1925]), 34–35. https://thenewcriterion1926.files.wordpress.com/2014/12/woolf-on-being-ill.pdf, accessed on May 23 2022.
2 In recent times, Paul Kalanithi's end of life memoir and less well-known Tom Lubbock's published diaries, both works posthumously published, are enlightening examples in this instance. See Paul Kalanithi, *When Breath Becomes Air* (London: Random House Publishing Group, 2016), and Tom Lubbock, *Until Further Notice I am Alive* (London: Granta Books), 2014.
3 G. S. Bowman, 'Emotions and Illness,' *Journal of Advanced Nursing* 34:2 (April 2001): 256–63, https://doi.org/10.1046/j.1365-2648.2001.01752.x.

https://doi.org/10.1515/9783110731002-005

as an encounter between past individual experiences, medical interventions or lack thereof, and cultural and political definitions of illness: this emotional encounter, it is argued, is 'complex, difficult to render in words, frayed at the edges, messy at its core, political through and through.'[4] How can we possibly capture what it feels like to be ill or fear illness? This is the overarching question that our essay contributes to through the analysis of mental health patients' responses. Our methodology mirrors the complexity of the emotional aspects of experiencing illness: through our open-ended questionnaire, we treat the covid-19 pandemic as a collective event that sits at the border of biology and society, and medicine and history. As will become apparent in the course of the essay, by exploring the emotional life of the coronavirus, we seek, as Boddice and Hitzer also write, to 'collapse the distinction between biology and culture,'[5] namely to suggest that sociocultural processes are inscribed on the body at the same time as the body commands and forms these same processes. As will be seen here, this becomes especially apparent in the case of epidemics and pandemics.

With regard to the 2020 pandemic, emotions such as fear and anger were documented as mediators between the public and various governmental bodies;[6] fear in particular was seen as affecting key survival mechanisms such as decision readiness, deliberation, information acquisition, risk perception, and thinking;[7] while during the latest stages of the pandemic only few emotional upregulation strategies such as 'savouring the moment' appeared to increase changes towards joy.[8] Overall, fear, uncertainty, anxiety, and depression were the most oft-cited emotions associated with at least the first pandemic year's stages.[9] Despite the several studies examining emotional responses to the pandemic, none have started unpacking the workings of the emotional resilience in the pandemic years. This is our immediate objective in the present study: how do emotions enable individuals to construct

---

4 Rob Boddice and Bettina Hitzer, *Feeling Dis-Ease in Modern History: Experiencing Medicine and Illness* (Bloomsbury Publishing, 2022), 2.

5 Boddice and Hitzer, *Feeling Dis-Ease in Modern History*, 3.

6 Emma A. Renström and Hanna Bäck, 'Emotions During The Covid-19 Pandemic: Fear, Anxiety, And Anger As Mediators Between Threats And Policy Support And Political Actions,' *Journal of Applied Social Psychology* 51:8 (2021): 861–77, https://doi.org/10.1111/jasp.12806.

7 Peter Huang, 'Pandemic Emotions: The Good, The Bad, and The Unconscious —Implications for Public Health, Financial Economics, Law, and Leadership,' *Northwestern Journal of Law & Social Policy* 16:2 (2021): 81.

8 Iris Schelhorn et al., 'Emotions and Emotion Up-Regulation during the COVID-19 Pandemic in Germany,' *PLOS ONE* 17:1 (2022): e0262283, https://doi.org/10.1371/journal.pone.0262283.

9 Ana Luisa Pedrosa et al., 'Emotional, Behavioral, and Psychological Impact of the COVID–19 Pandemic,' *Frontiers in Psychology* 11 (2020), https://doi.org/10.3389/fpsyg.2020.566212.

resilient strategies through the current pandemic, and how do these emotions and strategies relate to previous epidemics and pandemics?

A key aspect of the emotional experience of illness that has been well-documented is its relationship with narrative: 'Narrative knowledge is what one uses to understand the meaning and significance of stories through cognitive, symbolic, and affective means.'[10] In the case of the Covid-19 pandemic, emotions showed a specific narrative arc whose protagonists were primarily the emotions of fear, anger, and ultimately acceptance. For example, when perceived with a threat, people are more likely to seek for help, communicate their problem, look for emotional support and try to self-regulate their emotions. These coping mechanisms in turn make one accept a difficult situation and achieve resilience. However, it is outmost importance to acknowledge that a person that may be under stress, accepts negative emotions and then be willing to affectively cope with them. By being open to this truth, people are more likely to show self-compassion and empathy that will eventually build their emotional resilience. This is also evident by the success of narrative therapy for building resilience. Narrative therapy is the process of helping people to overcome problems through engaging in therapeutic dialogs. Research has shown that by sharing traumatic life events, the process of communication is facilitated, a key characteristic of resilience, and helps people rewrite a traumatic experience, in a more self-improving narrative.[11]

It is without doubt that the outbreak of the Covid-19 pandemic, and the lock-down implementations specifically, increased psychological distress and resulted in an elevation of psychological conditions such as anxiety and depression.[12] However, research suggests that experiencing both positive and negative emotions during traumatic events is associated with self-protective behaviors that build resilience. Moreover, research has found that positive emotions significantly moderated depression and anxiety symptoms, during the Covid-19 pandemic. Having established positive emotions during a crisis, people are more likely to express gratitude, love, optimism, and contentment, which have shown to promote resilience.[13] Enhancing resilience has been associated with better

---

10 Arnstein Finset, 'Emotions, Narratives and Empathy in Clinical Communication,' *International Journal of Integrated Care* 10:5 (2010): 53, https://doi.org/10.5334/ijic.490.

11 Mahdis Ghandehari et al, 'The Effect Of Narrative Therapy On Resiliency Of Women Who Have Referred To Counseling Centers In Isfahan,' *International Journal of Education & Psychology Researchers* 4:65–70 (2018), https://DOI.org/10.4103/2395-2296.204124.

12 Sijia Li et al., 'The Impact of COVID-19 Epidemic Declaration on Psychological Consequences: A Study on Active Weibo Users', *International Journal of Environmental Research and Public Health* 17:6 (January 2020): 2032, https://doi.org/10.3390/ijerph17062032.

13 Martin E. P. Seligman, *Flourish: A Visionary New Understanding of Happiness and Well-Being* (New York, NY, US: Free Press, 2011).

mental wellbeing, along with improvements in psychological outcomes such as self-efficacy, positive emotion, and coping.[14] Similar results have been observed during previous crisis, like the SARS epidemic. Interestingly, longitudinal studies have shown that people at the time were extremely fearful of the disease and reported adverse psychological distress, due to high mortality rate and no vaccine nor treatment have been found. As a result, psychologists developed an alternative debriefing model called Strength-Focused and Meaning-Oriented Approach for Resilience and Transformation (SMART), designed to promote resilience. During these debriefing sessions, participants have to recognize the interconnectedness of their emotions and reflect on their negative emotions. Results for this model were quite successful, as symptoms of depression significantly reduced, even after the therapy was finished. These findings support the hypothesis that when dealing with negative emotions in a constructive way, stressful life events like natural disasters can promote lifetime resilience.

More particularly, Philip Strong's seminal study on 'epidemic psychology'[15] and the key role of emotional development were explicitly or implicitly confirmed through pandemic-related studies that showed the public's 'sense of shock and chaos; [. . .] gradual adjustment to the new reality; and [. . .] fears and concerns for themselves and loved ones' as the pandemic became an accepted reality.[16] Similarly, an analysis of 122M Twitter responses related to the pandemic and posted throughout the year 2020 showed that the three psycho-social phases of any epidemic as theorized by Strong were correlative with three key emotions, namely fear, then anger, and then acceptance:

In the refusal phase, users refused to accept reality despite the increasing number of deaths in other countries. In the anger phase (started after the announcement of the first death in the country), users' fear translated into anger about the looming feeling that things were about to change. Finally, in the acceptance phase, which began after the authorities imposed physical-distancing measures, users settled into a 'new normal' for their daily activities.[17]

---

14 Ji Hee Lee et al., 'Resilience: A Meta-Analytic Approach,' *Journal of Counseling & Development* 91:3 (2013): 269–79, https://doi.org/10.1002/j.1556-6676.2013.00095.x.

15 Philip Strong, 'Epidemic Psychology: A Model,' *Sociology of Health & Illness* 12:3 (1990): 249–59, https://doi.org/10.1111/1467-9566.ep11347150.

16 Inbar Levkovich and Shiri Shinan-Altman, 'Impact Of The COVID-19 Pandemic On Stress And Emotional Reactions In Israel: A Mixed-Methods Study,' *International Health*, 13:4 (October 13, 2020): 361, https://doi.org/10.1093/inthealth/ihaa081.

17 Luca Maria Aiello et al., 'How Epidemic Psychology Works on Twitter: Evolution of Responses to the COVID-19 Pandemic in the U.S.' *Humanities and Social Sciences Communications* 8:179 (2021): 1–15, https://doi.org/10.1057/s41599-021-00861-3.

Although Strong does not focus on the emotions of an epidemic or a pandemic themselves, but rather on the language sharing that accompanies emotional responses to a crisis, and that is characteristic of epidemic psychology, a plethora of many crucial emotions and affects are present through the experience of disease—So but when my father diedeither the actual experience or the expectant one. It appears then that, as Strong theorized regarding the HIV epidemic, there is a specific narrative arc through which individuals and communities go through during an epidemic or a pandemic: 'collective social psychology has its own epidemic form, can be activated by other crises besides those of disease and is rooted in the fundamental properties of language and human interaction.'[18] This human interaction, the narratives engendered by individuals trying to navigate the Covid-19 threat, and their emotional resilience strategies have recently been argued to contain 'therapeutic value,' to 'advance collective knowledge and understanding meaningfully,' and even to contain 'potentially foundational contributions to extant biomedical knowledge.'[19] The emotions that underpin the relationship between collective narrative and individual resilience strategies are of interest to this essay.

In the last twenty years, with the rise of narrative medicine and the implementation of interdisciplinary approaches to illness and treatment, a number of emotions, and crucially, their narrativization, have been proven to influence illness's experience and even outcomes.[20] Not only does narrativization of traumatic events

---

18 Strong, 'Epidemic Psychology,' 249.

19 Deepika Bahri, 'Why Stories about Illness Matter,' *The Lancet* 399, 10340 (2022): 2009–10, https://doi.org/10.1016/S0140–6736(22)00933–3.

20 Research in 1990 concluded that 'both the sociology of emotions and health and illness need to incorporate the concept of the living, embodied human subject and recent studies in bio-psycho-social research into their discourses. A focus on the emotionally expressive, embodied subject, who is active in the context of power and social control, can provide a useful approach for studying distressful feelings, society, and health' (Freund, Peter E. S. 'The Expressive Body: A Common Ground for the Sociology of Emotions and Health and Illness,' *Sociology of Health & Illness* 12:4 (1990): 452–77, https://doi.org/10.1111/1467-9566.ep11340419). Bowman's seminal research in 2001 contended that 'emotional reaction to illness is normal and that emotions expressed are likely to hold clues to individual adaptation' (Bowman, G. S. 'Emotions and Illness,' *Journal of Advanced Nursing,* 34:2 (2001): 256–63, https://doi.org/10.1046/j.1365-2648.2001.01752.x); Levenson's 2019 study examines the relationship between stress-specific emotions particular health outcomes (Levenson, Robert W. 'Stress and Illness: A Role for Specific Emotions,' *Psychosomatic Medicine* 81:8 (2019): 720–30, https://doi.org/10.1097/PSY.0000000000000736). In 2021, emotions such as vulnerability, sadness, and fear were established as playing 'a role in health maintenance or disease development' (Guimond, Anne-Josée, Laura D. Kubzansky, and Lewina O. Lee. 'Emotion and Illness,' in *Emotion in the Clinical Encounter*, edited by Rachel Schwartz, Judith A. Hall, and Lars G. Osterberg (New York, NY: McGraw Hill, 2021).

'serve [. . .] a healing as well as a heuristic function,'[21] it also helps bridge individual experiences with collective and historical events. Among the ever-present socio-political issues that the coronavirus pandemic laid bare, such as persistent inequality and modes of ill-governance, there is yet another aspect of living through a pandemic that painfully resonates with the past: the straining of individual and collective mental health under global illness. Time and again, safeguarding our bodies from infectious disease has inevitably placed our mental health at risk, with stress, burnout, depression, and post-traumatic stress disorder forming the ubiquitous lexicon of infectious disease's psychopathology.[22] Beyond the labelling of the psychopathological paradigm, however, the experience of living through a pandemic triggers certain emotional responses that are placed in a narrative arc, much like the emotional stages of grief. Indeed, as has been recently argued, 'emotion shares with narrative the basic temporal structure:'[23]

> Because emotions react to and evaluate events, to understand them we need to understand the sequence of events and their implications. I argue that this requires a narrative format. It allows making sense of emotions and communicating them. The narrative format requires spelling out the relevant background which is necessary to understand the meaning of events for a given individual, it relates the events, and it allows to transport, to interpret and to evaluate anew the events. Therefore the emotion process has a narrative quality. And narrating the emotional experiences has the power to transform them and the emotions they engender.[24]

Considering, as has been argued, that a person's 'macronarratives' are necessary for dealing with moments of crisis,[25] the exploration of the triptych of emotion, narrative, resilience can be fruitful to understand responses of individuals under duress. While it is apparent from Strong's theorization (and the more recent research projects' analyses) that the narrative/emotional arc experienced concurrently with illness, epidemic, or crisis is part of the process of coping, an analysis of how these and other emotions and affective states contribute to or impede individual resilience has not been conducted.

---

21 Robert Neimeyer and Heidi Levitt, 'Coping and Coherence: A Narrative Perspective on Resilience,' in *Coping with Stress: Effective People and Processes*, ed. C.R. Snyder (New York: Oxford Academic, 2001), 64.
22 Deepika Bahri, 'Why Stories about Illness Matter,' *The Lancet* 399, 10340 (May 28, 2022): 2009–10, https://doi.org/10.1016/S0140–6736(22)00933–3.
23 Tilmann Habermas, *Emotion and Narrative: Perspectives in Autobiographical Storytelling* (Cambridge University Press, 2019), 2.
24 Habermas, *Emotion and Narrative*, 2.
25 Neimeyer and Levitt, 'Coping and Coherence,' 49.

To this effect, for this study, we asked twenty individuals who had sought mental health support to provide their insights on the pandemic experience, in order to examine pandemic-related emotions and the ways through which they contributed to narratives of resilience. The question that we sought to answer is: how do emotional responses influence the resilience of individuals who are already diagnosed with mental health issues? In this essay, we present some preliminary findings on emotional responses and their relationship to individual resilience, attempting to contextualize and historize them according to established research on illness and emotion. Our findings are not meant to be representative of a particular group, but rather to be one starting point for analyses and theorizations of resilience at times of illness based on less quantifiable emotions.

Methodology

We devised a questionnaire, posing a series of open-ended questions written in Greek to individuals for whom one of the authors of the present essay has been acting as a therapist, due to relational difficulties, mental health issues, or their interest in psychological growth and well being. Twenty individuals living in Greece but also abroad were given a set of written questions and a week to return the questionnaire to their therapist, with the option of completing as many or as few questions as they wished. Ideally, the interviews would have been conducted face to face. However, pandemic restrictions at the time, and increased anxiety on the part of the participants, led us to collect the data in such a way. The answers were given handwritten to the authors of this essay, and have been translated from Greek to English by them. We disseminated the questionnaire to all adults who were being treated by the author/therapist at the private clinic, remotely or in person, regardless of their age, gender, sexual orientation, or race. Consent to participate was obtained after the process of research was explained to each prospective participant by their therapist. The participants of the study are here represented by random initials.

Through this method, we consciously sought to record collective responses to resilience during the pandemic. This is a tricky, and to an extent rightfully so, demonized aspect of studying emotion. As Boddice and Hitzer ask, 'Does a collective awareness or apprehension of smallpox amount to a community?'[26] In the same vein, does experiencing the Covid-19 pandemic across the same country mean

---

26 Boddice and Hitzer, *Feeling Dis-Ease*, 6.

one belongs to a singular emotional community? The answer that Boddice and Hitzer give is definite: it is during periods of collective crisis and 'widespread fear that we see the typical components of what is usually understood as community fall apart, and yet the collective is, nevertheless, experiencing something together, in common to a certain extent.'[27] By closely examining the responses of twenty individuals we sought not to collapse the biocultural differences of the individuals, but instead to focus on the shared aspects of the experience.

For this project, we employed of a combination of narrative medicine's definitive method, namely close-reading and the methodology known as the Listening Guide Method of Psychological Inquiry,[28] a discovery-based qualitative component that has been employed to delineate strategies for survival evidenced in the lives of the long-term survivors.[29] On the one hand, close-reading enables 'relationship-building among learners and individual awareness of the interior processes of the reader' as well as promoting 'justice in healthcare, participatory practice, egalitarian learning, and deep relationships in practice.'[30] On the other hand, the Listening Guide, inspired both by Rita Charon's use of close-reading in medical practice but also from psychiatrist Jonathan Shay's work with Vietnam War veterans, asks questions with a view to discover what can be learned from individuals' respective experiences and not with the ambition of categorizing them into psychological slots. Our study's questions are underpinned by the Listening Guide's four premises/overall questions:

Who is speaking and to whom?
In what body or physical space?
Telling what stories about which relationships?
In what societal and cultural frameworks?[31]

Lastly, the selected method was specifically chosen as the participants already had a relationship of trust with one of the authors of the present essay, which can

---

27 Boddice and Hitzer, *Feeling Dis–Ease*, 6–7.
28 Carol Gilligan et al., 'On the Listening Guide: A Voice-Centered Relational Method,' in *Qualitative Research in Psychology: Expanding Perspectives in Methodology and Design*, eds. Paul. M. Camic, Jean. E. Rhodes, and Lucy Yardley (Washington, DC, US: American Psychological Association, 2003), 157–72, https://doi.org/10.1037/10595-009.
29 Carol Gilligan and Jessica Eddy, 'Listening as a Path to Psychological Discovery: An Introduction to the Listening Guide,' *Perspectives on Medical Education* 6:2 (2017): 76–81, https://doi.org/10.1007/s40037-017-0335-3.
30 Rita Charon, *Close Reading: The Signature Method of Narrative Medicine, The Principles and Practice of Narrative Medicine* (Oxford University Press), https://oxfordmedicine.com/view/10.1093/med/9780199360192.001.0001/med-9780199360192-chapter-8, accessed 29 April 2022.
31 Gilligan and Eddy, 'Listening as a Path,' 77.

further foster the Listening Guide's aspiration for 'authentic relationship and responsive listening [to] become integral to the process of discovery.'[32]

The questionnaire that the participants were asked to complete within a week contained the following open-ended questions:

1. How has the crisis of the pandemic influenced your mental health?
2. Which emotions did you experience during the two years of the pandemic?
3. Are there any emotions from past difficult experiences that resurfaced during the pandemic?
4. What does the term emotional resilience mean to you?
5. What kind of experiences do you think fortify a person's emotional resilience?
6. What kind of experiences do you think damage a person's emotional resilience?
7. Try to recall events that occurred during the pandemic, and the ways through which you persuaded/enabled yourself to handle them. How did you cope? Through which strategies? What stopped you from coping?
8. Do you consider yourself an easily adaptable person?
9. Do you consider yourself as someone who problem-solves? Who do you turn to when you need help?
10. What would you say you learnt, if anything, through the experience of the pandemic?

Results and Discussion: Defining Emotional Resilience through Narrative

Resilience is a concept lamented for its indefinability. As Andre Cavalcante writes, 'practices of resilient reception are multiple, diverse, and at times morally and politically ambiguous. They have no inherent nature.'[33] As a psychological construct, resilience has created a new market of self-care, while at the same time the discourse of resilience has often been shamelessly capitalized on by the State. The upshot of this, Mark Neocleous writes, is that resilience has become 'a new fetish' in the twenty-first century, and 'is central not only to the self-help industry, but also to the wider 'happiness studies' now being peddled by politicians and academic disciplines such as psychology and eco nomics [sic].'[34] The state demand to endure by improving the self comes in direct juxtaposition to resisting the

---

32 Gilligan and Eddy, 'Listening as a Path,' 80.

33 Andre Cavalcante, *Struggling for Ordinary: Media and Transgender Belonging in Everyday Life* (NYU Press, 2018), 130.

34 Mark Neocleous, 'Resisting Resilience,' *Radical Philosophy* 178 (2013), 5, https://www.radicalphilosophy.com/commentary/resisting-resilience, accessed 13 April 2023.

reproduction of inequality, it would seem. Whereas this is certainly true in many cases, it connotes a passive definition of resilience. As has been noted though, a resilient structure is 'more than simply sustainable,' it is primarily 'regenerative and diverse, relying not only on the capacity to absorb shocks like the popped housing bubble or the rising sea level, but to evolve with them,'[35] and, as we hope to argue here, critique as well. Therefore, we support the view that whereas the ability to be resilient is not necessarily a marker of 'healthy' human adaptation, or moral virtue,'[36] this ability, and its attendant emotions can provide fertile ground for criticizing existing systemic practices.

As part of our study, we asked all participants to describe what resilience means to each of them. Most of them related resilience to overcoming their own personal obstacles. This included managing and overcoming challenges posed on a global or national scale as well, challenges that complicated personal goals and seemed inescapable. Almost all of the participants recorded both positive and negative effects of the pandemic on their emotional state and their capability for resilience and adaptation. For example, more time at home and sharing ordinary experiences with loved ones on a daily basis were at the top of the positives for most participants, while the lack of choices and the lockdown constraints that were becoming more and more burdensome were described by the majority of the participants as the issue that caused the most negative pressure. Two of the participants characterized certain experiences in their lives as affected by the pandemic as both 'interesting and challenging,' thus exhibiting oxymoronic signs, which, as Boris Cyrulnik has argued, are 'characteristic of a personality that has been wounded but which still resists, that suffers but is happy enough to go on hoping despite everything.'[37] This is a view that was echoed by most participants. Another participant stated that 'personal and work [. . .] difficulties wear you down but also steel you' (T, 51), while a woman aged 20 answered the question 'What kind of experiences do you think fortify a person's emotional resilience?' by stating that 'some circumstances such as losing a loved one can fortify one's emotional resilience' (A).

Connecting the experience of the pandemic to previous traumatic circumstances (such as the compulsory military service in Greece, according to T) and to the experience of losing loved ones frequently appeared in participants' answers. When they were called to answer the question 'Are there any emotions from past

---

35 Jamais Cascio, 'The Next Big Thing: Resilience,' *Foreign Policy* (blog), 28 September 2009, 92, https://foreignpolicy.com/2009/09/28/the-next-big-thing-resilience/, accessed 13 April 2023.

36 Cavalcante, *Struggling*, 130.

37 Boris Cyrulnik, 'Narrative Resilience: Neurological and Psychotherapeutic Reflections,' in *Multisystemic Resilience*, ed Michael Ungar (New York: Oxford University Press, 2021), 22.

difficult experiences that resurfaced during the pandemic?' their answers were compelling. 'Of course,' wrote 76-year-old N, 'I was grieving, in a sense, like when I lost my partner. The same old feeling of loneliness came back. I relived the sadness and fear that I had previously lived through in difficult times.' This is consistent with the testimonies found in past ethnographies around illness, most notably Perry Halkitis's 2014 study on survivors of AIDS and their narratives of resilience, where a small group of participants were asked questions on what triggered AIDS-related responses, with many of them answering that it was unrelated deaths that brought back emotions of illness for them. In particular, one AIDS generation study participant describes being emotionally triggered by his father's funeral, who died of pneumonia:

> So but when my father died, I think I had convinced myself that I had packed away a lot of—of my feelings and—and sadness and the trauma [. . .] I would go out to the parking lot because I was by myself sitting in the car, it would just erupt. Not for my father but all the memories. They only just scratched the surface, and they would come flooding back.[38]

In this participant's testimony, the father's death is what brings back traumatic memories of the epidemic, as opposed to N's reliving of her spouse's death through the traumatic isolation of Covid-19. It is interesting to note the similar verbal expression in participants of the present as well as Halkitis's study. Encountering the past through a current difficulty and reliving a past trauma is key for both these testimonies, and speaks to Halkitis's point that through the concurrent experience of individual and collective trauma, such experiences become normalized, thus leading to emotional resilience.[39]

This interweaving of emotions belonging to personal narrative and collective crisis appears to be at the heart of telling the story of resilience. Overall, 'researchers in the field of psychological resilience studies have only begun to shed light on the important role of narration as the central coping strategy or healing mechanism.'[40] On the one hand, resilience for the participants was seen as 'an

---

38 Perry N. Halkitis, *The AIDS Generation: Stories of Survival and Resilience* (New York: Oxford University Press, 2014), 90. In the same study, and within a US context, Halkitis also mentions that "aging HIV-positive men, those who are members of the AIDS generation, experience post-traumatic stress disorder (PTSD) at higher rates than even those who witnessed the event of 9/11 or any other disaster" (2014, 90). This is crucial for how we view epidemic and pandemic illnesses.
39 Halkitis, *The AIDS Generation*, 90.
40 Michael Basseler, 'Stories of Dangerous Life in the Post-Trauma Age: Toward a Cultural Narratology of Resilience,' in *Narrative in Culture*, ed. Astrid Erll and Roy Sommer (Berlin: De Gruyter, 2019), 19.

ongoing struggle to create and sustain the new normal that comes from recognition that life cannot be the same as it was before.'[41] More importantly, though, it is proven, as has been noted with regard to transgender resilience, that 'practices of resilient reception are, at base, survival strategies enacted as pragmatic responses to the powerfully affective encounters individuals have with media and society in the everyday.'[42] Time and again, the participants compared and contrasted their own experience of the pandemic with the narrative presented by the media and by people around them. To the question 'Which emotions did you experience during the two years of the pandemic?' 51-year-old, male, T answered: 'Anger for fake news and the silly theories that circulated at the time. Rage towards familiar and unfamiliar people who were taking absurd rumors seriously.' Similarly, 76-year-old, female N. writes of her need to constantly be 'informed,' so that she could 'process external data in order to draw conclusions and prioritize [her] needs.'

This speaks to the special relationship between resilience and narrative, both personal and collective. Cyrulnik provides some helpful first insights in this regard. As he explains in his book *Resilience: How Your Inner Strength Can Set You Free from the Past*, 'what we are at any given moment obliges us to use our ecological, emotional, and verbal environments to 'knit' ourselves. We might feel that, if a single stitch is dropped, everything will unravel, but in fact, if just one stitch holds, we can start all over again.'[43] Similarly, as Neimeyer and Levitt argue, resilience arises

> from the double effort first to describe our coping responses in the micronarratives of our life story, and then to inscribe these as personal resources in the more or less coherent macronarratives that consolidate our sense of identity over time. 'Coping' then becomes a storied construction, created and sustained within a distinctively human meaning-making process.[44]

What became apparent through this study is that the emotional experience of the pandemic was for the participants an opportunity to combine their micronarratives and the macronarratives, even as their personal experience differed from what they heard on the news. For many of the participants, a crucial emotion

41 Patrice Buzzanell and S. Shenoy-Packer, 'How Resilience Is Constructed in Everyday Work-Life Experience Across the Lifespan,' in *Communicating Hope and Resilience Across the Lifespan*, eds Gary Beck and Thomas Socha (New York: Peter Lang Verlag, 2015), 150, https://doi.org/10.3726/978-1-4539-1520-2.

42 Cavalcante, *Struggling*, 130.

43 Boris Cyrulnik, *Resilience: How Your Inner Strength Can Set You Free from the Past* (Penguin, 2011), 13.

44 Neimeyer and Heidi Levitt, 'Coping and Coherence,' 64.

was that of patience, which in turn enabled them to feel a sense of belonging to a wider community of people. This may shed new light not only on how illness and the fear of illness is perceived by a collective, but also on ways to methodologically address the separate, yet collective experience of illness-related emotions.

Answering the question 'What would you say you learnt, if anything, through the experience of the pandemic?' T answered that he learnt to look at the world as 'a totality:' 'You are not the centre of the world, other people suffer as well [. . .] humility, calm, solidarity [are necessary].' Similarly, 76-year-old M responded that she learnt how to express empathy and solidarity. Such findings confirm the suggestion that resilience is often conceived as a 'narrative project' (Basseler 2019, 22), one of a collaborative nature at that. What went against dominant literature surrounding resilience and narrative is the fact that the conflict between micro- and macronarratives seemed to enhance participants' resilience, which according to Cyrulnik should not be possible:

> When the injured person's story is consistent with the surrounding stories, the person experiences a sense of calm that regulates brain function. But when the intimate and collective stories are conflicting, the maladjusted casualty feels isolated and misunderstood, making the process of resilience difficult.[45]

On the contrary, we noted that the individuals in our study largely sought strength in precisely such conflicts. More than half of the participants wrote that they derive their resilience from a combination of adapting while simultaneously sticking to their goals, even when the 'surrounding atmosphere, the sociopolitical and financial circumstances are against me' (P).

Lastly, we notice that even though the participants of the study had at the time of providing their answers not gone through Covid-19, or else chose not to disclose it, the emotions that they describe are similar to testimonials provided by survivors of the Ebola virus. Specifically, in a 2003 study of Ebola in Uganda, eleven participants described their experience of surviving Ebola as 'an escape into peaceful awareness, hope for a world outside of fear, persistence in defying death, and a constant fear of dying.'[46] To the question 'What would you say you learnt, if anything, through the experience of the pandemic?' the responses were mostly hopeful. 'I appreciated the resilience of our culture,' responded T, and learned to show 'peaceful humility;' N responded with 'empathy and solidarity;' S wrote that the constant fear of illness taught him how to 'patiently wait for the

---

45 Cyrulnik, 'Narrative Resilience.'

46 Rozzano Locsin et al., 'Surviving Ebola: Understanding Experience through Artistic Expression', *International Nursing Review* 50 (October 1, 2003): 156–66, 1, https://doi.org/10.1046/j.1466-7657.2003.00194.x.

darkness to leave our planet;' and S contended that although he was surprised by the constant 'fear at mine and others' death,' he also learnt to be 'hopeful' for the future once the pandemic would be over.

Limitations

Although this might be limiting in the sense that pauses, and other verbal expressions cannot be part of the data under examination, the written responses that we assume were compiled over some time provided the participants with time to reflect on their answers, and the writers of this essay with ideal material to close-read.

Conclusion

The findings of our small study mostly confirmed that emotional resilience exists in-between one's personal narrative and its correspondence to the micronarrative, without though this meaning that the two narratives must be in complete accordance. The emotions recorded by the participants (loneliness, fear, patience, reliving of trauma, and hopefulness) are consistent with the narrative of the epidemic provided by Strong and others. A significant addition to this narrative (and slightly unexpected if one considers the isolating and alienating ramifications of social distancing, which was long and repeated in Greece) was the emotion of empathy, which seemed to be pervading in most accounts. Thus, the relationship between resilience and empathy, especially in the framework of illness, would be fruitful research for the future.

References

Aiello, Luca Maria., Daniele Quercia, Ke Zhou, Marios Constantinides, Sanja Šćepanović, and Sagar Joglekar. 'How Epidemic Psychology Works on Twitter: Evolution of Responses to the COVID-19 Pandemic in the U.S.' *Humanities and Social Sciences Communications* 8:1 (2021): 1–15. https://doi. org/10.1057/s41599-021-00861-3.

Bahri, Deepika. 'Why Stories about Illness Matter;' *The Lancet* 399:10340 (2022): 2009–10. https://doi. org/10.1016/S0140-6736(22)00933-3.

Basseler, Michael. 'Stories of Dangerous Life in the Post-Trauma Age: Toward a Cultural Narratology of Resilience;' In *Narrative in Culture*, eds. Astrid Erll and Roy Sommer, 15–36. Berlin: De Gruyter, 2019.

Boddice, Rob, and Bettina Hitzer. *Feeling Dis-Ease in Modern History: Experiencing Medicine and Illness*. London: Bloomsbury Publishing, 2022.

Bowman, G. S. 'Emotions and Illness.' *Journal of Advanced Nursing* 34:2 (2001): 256–63. https://doi.org/10.1046/j.1365-2648.2001.01752.x.

Buzzanell, Patrice and S. Shenoy-Packer. 'How Resilience Is Constructed in Everyday Work-Life Experience Across the Lifespan.' in *Communicating Hope and Resilience Across the Lifespan*, ed. Gary A. Beck and Thomas Socha, 138–55. New York: Peter Lang, 2014.

Cascio, Jamais. 'The Next Big Thing: Resilience.' *Foreign Policy* (blog), 28 September 2009. https://foreignpolicy.com/2009/09/28/the-next-big-thing-resilience/.

Cavalcante, Andre. *Struggling for Ordinary: Media and Transgender Belonging in Everyday Life*. New York: NYU Press, 2018.

Charon, Rita. *Close Reading: The Signature Method of Narrative Medicine. The Principles and Practice of Narrative Medicine*. Oxford University Press, 2016. https://oxfordmedicine.com/view/10.1093/med/9780199360192.001.0001/med-9780199360192-chapter-8. Accessed 29 April 2022.

Cyrulnik, Boris. 'Narrative Resilience: Neurological and Psychotherapeutic Reflections.' In *Multisystemic Resilience: Adaptation and Transformation in Contexts of Change*, ed. Michael Ungar, 100–110. New York: Oxford University Press, 2021. https://doi.org/10.1093/oso/9780190095888.003.0006.

Cyrulnik, Boris. *Resilience: How Your Inner Strength Can Set You Free from the Past*. New York: J.P. Tarcher/ Penguin, 2011.

Finset, Arnstein. 'Emotions, Narratives and Empathy in Clinical Communication.' *International Journal of Integrated Care* 10:5 (2010) https://doi.org/10.5334/ijic.490.

Freund, Peter E. S. 'The Expressive Body: A Common Ground for the Sociology of Emotions and Health and Illness.' *Sociology of Health & Illness* 12:4 (1990): 452–77. https://doi.org/10.1111/1467-9566.ep11340419.

Ghandehari, Mahdis, and Leila Moosavi, Fatemeh Rasooli Jazi, Mozhgan Arefi and Soodabeh Ahmadzadeh. 'The Effect of Narrative Therapy on Resiliency of Women Who Have Referred to Counseling Centers in Isfahan.' *International Journal of Education & Psychology Researchers* 4:2 (2018): 65–70. https://doi.org/10.4103/2395-2296.204124

Gilligan, Carol, and Jessica Eddy. 'Listening as a Path to Psychological Discovery: An Introduction to the Listening Guide.' *Perspectives on Medical Education* 6:2 (2017): 76–81. https://doi.org/10.1007/s40037-017-0335-3.

Gilligan, Carol., Renée Spencer, M. Katherine Weinberg and Tatiana Bertsch. 'On the Listening Guide: A Voice-Centered Relational Method.' In *Qualitative Research in Psychology: Expanding Perspectives in Methodology and Design*, edited by Paul. M. Camic, Jean. E. Rhodes and Lucy Yardley, 157–72. Washington, DC, US: American Psychological Association, 2003. https://doi.org/10.1037/10595-009.

Guimond, Anne-Josée, Laura D. Kubzansky, and Lewina O. Lee. 'Emotion and Illness.' In *Emotion in the Clinical Encounter*, edited by Rachel Schwartz, Judith A.Hall, and Lars G. Osterberg. New York, NY: McGraw Hill, 2021.

Habermas, Tilmann. *Emotion and Narrative: Perspectives in Autobiographical Storytelling*. Cambridge: Cambridge University Press, 2019. https://doi.org/10.1017/9781139424615.

Halkitis, Perry N. *The AIDS Generation: Stories of Survival and Resilience*. New York: Oxford University Press, 2014. https://archive.org/details/aidsgenerationst0000halk

Huang, Peter. 'Pandemic Emotions: The Good, The Bad, and The Unconscious – Implications for Public Health, Financial Economics, Law, and Leadership.' *Northwestern Journal of Law & Social Policy* 16:2 (2021): 80–129.

Kalanithi, Paul. *When Breath Becomes Air*. New York: Random House Publishing Group, 2016.

Lee, Ji Hee., Suk Kyung Nam, A-Reum Kim, Boram Kim, Min Young Lee and Sang Min Lee. "Resilience: A Meta-Analytic Approach." *Journal of Counseling & Development* 91:3 (2013): 269–79. https://doi. org/10.1002/j.1556-6676.2013.00095.x.

Levenson, Robert W. 'Stress and Illness: A Role for Specific Emotions.' *Psychosomatic Medicine* 81:8 (October 2019): 720–30. https://doi.org/10.1097/PSY.0000000000000736.

Levkovich, Inbar and Shiri Shinan-Altman. 'Impact of the COVID-19 Pandemic on Stress and Emotional Reactions in Israel: A Mixed-Methods Study.' *International Health* 13:4 (2020). https://doi.org/10.1093/inthealth/ihaa081.

Li, Sijia., Yilin Wang, Jia Xue, Nan Zhao and Tingshao Zhu. "The Impact of COVID-19 Epidemic Declaration on Psychological Consequences: A Study on Active Weibo Users." *International Journal of Environmental Research and Public Health* 17:6 (2020): 2032. https://doi.org/10.3390/ijerph17062032.

Locsin, Rozzano., Alan Barnard, Gerald Matua, and Bongomin Bodo. "Surviving Ebola: Understanding Experience through Artistic Expression." *International Nursing Review* 50 (2003): 156–66. https://doi.org/10.1046/j.1466-7657.2003.00194.x.

Lubbock, Tom. *Until Further Notice, I am Alive*. London: Granta Books, 2014.

Neimeyer, Robert, and Heidi Levitt. 'Coping and Coherence: A Narrative Perspective on Resilience.' In *Coping with Stress: Effective People and Processes*, edited by C.R. Snyder, 47–67. New York: Oxford Academic, 2001.

Neocleous, Mark. "Resisting Resilience." *Radical Philosophy* 178 (2013). https://www.radicalphiloso phy.com/commentary/resisting-resilience. Accessed 13 April 2023.

Pedrosa, Ana Luisa., Letícia Bitencourt, Ana Cláudia Fontoura Fróes, Maria Luíza Barreto Cazumbá, Ramon Gustavo Bernardino Campos, Stephanie Bruna Camilo Soares de Brito, and Ana Cristina Simões e Silva. 'Emotional, Behavioral, and Psychological Impact of the COVID-19 Pandemic.' *Frontiers in Psychology* 11 (2020). https://doi.org/10.3389/fpsyg.2020.566212.

Renström, Emma A and Hanna Bäck. 'Emotions during the Covid-19 Pandemic: Fear, Anxiety, and Anger as Mediators between Threats and Policy Support and Political Actions.' *Journal of Applied Social Psychology* 51:8 (2021): 861–77. https://doi.org/10.1111/jasp.12806.

Seligman, Martin E. P. *Flourish: A Visionary New Understanding of Happiness and Well-Being*. New York; Free Press, 2011.

Schelhorn, Iris., Swantje Schlüter, Kerstin Paintner, Youssef Shiban, Ricardo Lugo, Marie Meyer and Stefan Sütterlin. 'Emotions and Emotion Up-Regulation during the COVID-19 Pandemic in Germany.' *PLOS ONE* 17:1 (2022): e0262283. https://doi.org/10.1371/journal.pone.0262283.

Strong, Philip. 'Epidemic Psychology: A Model.' *Sociology of Health & Illness* 12:3 (1990): 249–59. https://doi.org/10.1111/1467-9566.ep11347150.

Woolf, Virginia. *On Being Ill*. The Hogarth Press. 1930 [1925]. Accessed on May 23 2022. https://thenewcriterion1926.files.wordpress.com/2014/12/woolf-on-being-ill.pdf

Christopher Smith
Chapter Five
Covid-19, Myth, Memory and the Second World War

Introduction

The novel SARS-CoV-2 virus, which emerged in Wuhan, China, in late 2019, swept across the world in 2020. As of March 2022, the virus, and resulting disease, Covid-19, has killed approximately six million people.[1] In Britain, the disease struck particularly hard, deaths per million of the population numbering 2,578 at the time of writing. A figure comparable to, or higher than, many other economically developed European countries.[2] This tally came in spite of a highly successful vaccine roll-out programme, which has significantly reduced mortality and transmission in the UK. As was reported at the time, for much of the pandemic, Britain under-performed compared to similarly developed nations.[3]

The response of the British Conservative government to the pandemic was to implement highly stringent, invasive measures to diminish transmission, relieve pressure on healthcare infrastructure, and ultimately reduce mortality. These measures included the imposition of highly restrictive 'lockdowns' – rules, underpinned by legislation, restricting both movement and economic activity. The Prime Minister, Boris Johnson, outlined these extraordinary new rules in a letter sent to each household in the United Kingdom:

> we are giving one simple instruction – you **must** stay at home.
>
> You should not meet friends or relatives who do not live in your home. You may only leave your home for very limited purposes, such as buying food and medicine, exercising once a day and seeking medical attention. You can travel to and from work but should work from home if you can.
>
> When you do have to leave your home, you should ensure, wherever possible, that you are two metres apart from anyone outside of your household.

---

1 COVID-19 Excess Mortality Collaborators, 'Estimating Excess Mortality Due To The COVID-19 Pandemic: A Systematic Analysis Of COVID-19–Related Mortality, 2020–21,' *Lancet*, 399:10334 (2021), 1513–1536, https://doi.org/10.1016/S0140–6736(21)02796-3.
2 France stands at 2,245; Italy at 2,736; Spain at 2,247; and Germany at 1,633. Worldometer, 2022, https://www.worldometers.info/coronavirus/, accessed 13 May 2022.
3 Alexander Smith, 'Britain's Covid daily death toll is one of the worst in the world. What went wrong?' *NBC News*, 22 January 2021, https://www.nbcnews.com/news/world/britain-s-covid-daily-death-toll-one-worst-world-what-n1255261, accessed 24 May 2021.

https://doi.org/10.1515/9783110731002-006

These rules must be observed. So, if people break the rules, the police will issue fines and disperse gatherings.[4]

This has been widely viewed as the most extraordinary and invasive set of limitation on the basic freedoms of British citizens since the Second World War. *The Sunday Times* described this momentous decision in terms which directly referenced that conflict: 'Boris Johnson had ordered an expansion of the state not seen since the Second World War to save the National Health Service, an institution formed in the cauldron of that conflict.'[5] The article was accompanied with an illustration by Russel Herneman, Julian Osbaldstone and Tony Bell.[6] It depicted a couple sneaking to the pub stating, 'a swift half won't hurt', but with Boris Johnson sternly looking down on them, hands on his hips, in disapproval. The caption of the illustration reads, 'Careless Walk Costs Lives'. The cartoon was a direct homage to the Second World War's 'Careless Talk Costs Lives' posters, by the *Punch* cartoonist and later editor, (Cyril) Kenneth Bird who went by the penname Fougasse.[7]

The *Sunday Times* was hardly alone in framing its reporting of the Covid-19 crisis around the memory of the Second World War. Politicians, including the Prime Minister, Boris Johnson, were also keen to draw such comparisons. This chapter outlines some of the efforts by the British government and the print media to link the Covid-19 crisis to the British cultural memory of the war and how myths regarding that conflict were used as framing devices to explain or justify government policy.[8] In doing so, it demonstrates the perceived significance

---

4 Boris Johnson, 'Correspondence: Prime Minister Letter To Nation On Coronavirus', 28 March 2020, https://www.gov.uk/government/publications/pm-letter-to-nation-on-coronavirus, accessed 24 May 2021.
5 Tim Shipman and Caroline Wheeler, 'Ten Days That Shook Britain – And Changed The Nation For Ever; The Inside Story Of How Boris Johnson Changed His Priorities: Save Lives First, And Then Salvage The Economy,' *The Sunday Times*, 22 March 2020, 6, https://www.thetimes.co.uk/arti cle/coronavirus-ten-days-that-shook-britain-and-changed-the-nation-for-ever-spz6sc9vb, accessed 24 May 2021.
6 Russel Herneman, Julian Osbaldstone and Tony Bell, "Careless Walk Costs Lives," 22 March 2020, https://www.thetimes.co.uk/article/coronavirus-ten-days-that-shook-britain-and-changed-the-nation-for-ever-spz6sc9vb, accessed 24 May 2021.
7 Howard Coster, 'Bird, (Cyril) Kenneth [Fougasse] (1887–1965),' *Oxford Dictionary of National Bi-ography*, (Oxford: Oxford University Press, 2004), https://www.oxforddnb.com/view/10.1093/ref: odnb/9780198614128.001.0001/odnb-9780198614128-e-1002870, accessed 24 May 2021.
8 For over–views of Britain, myth and the war, see: Angus Calder, *The Myth of the Blitz* (London: Cape, 1991); Malcolm Smith, *Britain and 1940: History, Myth And Popular Memory* (London: Routledge 2000); Mark Connelly, *We can take It: Britain and the Memory of the Second World War* (Harlow: Pearson, 2004).

and legacies of the conflict in twenty-first century Britain and how the myths of the war continue to shape government and media rhetoric. But how effective have these efforts been? How readily has the British public accepted and drawn upon the comparisons made between the Covid-19 crisis and the Second World War? This chapter draws upon the *#RecordCovid19* project to test the reception of this messaging. It demonstrates that, at least in the case of the respondents to *#RecordCovid19* project, the Second World War has surprisingly little resonance. The project overwhelmingly received responses from young women. As such, it is possible that the relevance of the Second World War in British cultural memory is fading among this demographic.

Britain, Myth and The Second World War

That the national discourse surrounding Covid-19 crisis, which has led to the infection of over 22 million British citizens and resulted in the premature deaths of at least 176,708 people in the United Kingdom alone,[9] has been framed around the Second World War is not surprising. As Lucy Noakes and Juliette Pattinson have noted

> Few historical events have resonated as fully in modern British culture as the Second World War. Despite it receding further into the distant past with that generation's passing, it continues to have a lingering and very vivid presence in British popular culture so that even those born in its aftermath have particular 'memories' of it.[10]

These myths and memories have, in recent decades, become a core subject of interest to historians of Britain's wartime experience.[11] Various different myths of the conflict abound. Key to this chapter and the Covid-19 crisis are three key myths: the 'People's War'; Churchill as the 'man of destiny'; and the creation of a 'New Jerusalem'.

---

9 Worldometer, 2021, 'United Kingdom Coronavirus Cases,' https://www.worldometers.info/coronavirus/uk/, accessed 13 May 2022.
10 Lucy Noakes and Juliette Pattinson, 'Introduction: "Keep Calm and Carry On": The Cultural Memory of the Second World War in Britain,' in *British Cultural Memory and the Second World War*, ed. Lucy Noakes and Juliette Pattinson (London: Bloomsbury, 2014), 2.
11 Penny Summerfield, *Reconstructing Women's Wartime Lives: Discourse and Subjectivity in Oral Histories of the Second World War* (Manchester: Manchester University Press, 1997); Sonya O. Rose, *Which People's War?: National Identity and Citizenship in Wartime Britain 1939–1945* (Oxford: Oxford University Press, 2003); Noakes and Pattinson (eds.), *British Cultural Memory and the Second World War*.

In this context, a myth is not necessarily an event, or series of events, which did not happen. Instead, myth should be understood, in Roland Barthes analysis, as a purified picture of the past, which airbrushes out unfortunate or uncomfortable complexity from the desired narrative and gives historical actions 'the simplicity of their essences'.[12] To provide an example, in post-war France myths of 'resistancialism' emerged regarding the Vichy regime of 1940 to 1944: these minimised the collaboration, hardships and brutalities of the Vichy regime; promoted sites and groups associated with the French resistance; and associated the French nation with resistance.[13] Rather than engage with bitter and divisive analysis of those years, blighted by collaboration and atrocity, resistancialism offered a heroic interpretation of them in which Nazism was imposed on France and the French resisted. One of the central myths of the Second World War to emerge in Britain, was that the British were fighting a 'People's War'. That is, the existential threat posed by Nazi Germany, particularly in 1940, led the British public to come together in a spirit of unprecedented unity. Everyone did their bit be it on the front lines or on the Home front, they did so with the quintessentially British 'stiff upper lip', and in doing so the rifts between class and gender closed. Yet, this narrative over-states the extent of those changes and glosses over extent to which those fractures continued to persist.[14] Such myths were imposed from both "above", via government messaging and the media, and from "below" by the people themselves whose morale to which the government was in thrall. The state could only prosecute the war with the participation and acceptance of the people. As Angus Calder put it in 1969, were the people 'depressed by their conviction that victory would be the prelude to a new slump? Then plans must be made to ensure that life really would be better after the war'.[15]

Through created in the furnace of wartime, during the post-war period these myths of the Second World War have remained; always important and always present. This does not mean that they necessarily have remained static. For example, the People's War, originally a radical view of Britain's wartime experience, was somewhat diminished and changed in the Thatcherite 1980s. The idea of the united mass of Britons, in collective solidarity facing down existential thread of the Axis powers, was displaced and subordinated to a narrative of key heroes, Sir

12 Roland Barthes, *Myth Today*, in *Mythologies*, ed. Roland Barthes, selected and trans. by Annette Lavers (London: Vintage, [1957] 2009), 169–170.
13 Henry Rousso, *The Vichy Syndrome: History And Memory In France Since 1944*, trans. Arthur Goldhammer (Cambridge, MA: Harvard University Press, [1987] 1991), 10.
14 Penny Summerfield, 'Women, War and Social Change: Women in Britain in World War II,' in *Total War and Social Change*, ed. Arthur Marwick (London: Palgrave, 1988), 95–118.
15 Angus Calder, *The People's War: Britain, 1939–1945* (London: Pimlico, 1996).

Winston Churchill above all elevated to the 'man of destiny'. This view of the war was better suited the individualistic ideology of the government of the day and the decision by Margaret Thatcher to once again take Britain to war, following the Argentinian invasion of the Falkland Islands.[16] Mark Connelly describes this process as the placing of an increased 'emphasis on the image of Churchill and a desire to set the people free from interventionist controls.'[17]

Tied to the People's War myth, its natural conclusion in some ways, was the myth of the New Jerusalem. In the midst of the death, destruction and hardship, which had been visited on soldiers and civilians alike, a new Britain would be required after the war concluded. This would be a physical rebuilding of the nation, sweeping away destroyed, damaged or decrepit infrastructure and housing, replacing it with a modern, planned physical environment.[18] This was part of a wider, prevailing view that, hitherto, society had failed millions of its citizens, who had been left to the ravages of want, disease, ignorance, squalor and idleness.[19] After the British people had sacrificed so much to ensure victory, a consensus among the people and politicians emerged that it was incumbent on the postwar government to build a just, bountiful future. This would be the welfare state. As Lord Addison, the Leader of the Labour Party in the House of Lords, put it in 1944, 'We are not looking for (if I may so express it) a mushroom New Jerusalem, but we are looking for a determined and disinterested endeavour to apply the lessons of our great experiences, so that life and opportunity in our homeland shall be more worthy of the people who inhabit it.'[20] Arthur Marwick described such sentiment as the psychological impact of war, 'that such appalling slaughter must be for something'.[21] Tied to this idea is that the war produced a period of 'consensus' politics, which was in the view of Paul Addison saw all three major parties go 'to the polls in 1945 committed to principles of social and economic reconstruction' and this consensus was 'positive and purposeful'.[22] This general consensus broadly would hold firm until the Premiership of Margaret Thatcher. Yet,

---

16 Steven Fielding, Bill Schwartz and Richard Toye, *The Churchill Myths* (Oxford: Oxford University Press, 2022), 57.

17 Connelly, *We Can Take It*, 11.

18 John Stevenson, 'The New Jerusalem,' in *The Making of Britain: Echoes of Greatness*, ed. Lesley M. Smith (London: Macmillan Education Ltd., 1988), 53–70.

19 William H. B. Beveridge, *Social Insurance and Allied Services: Report by Sir William Beveridge* (London: HMSO, 1942), 170.

20 *Hansard*, Lords Debate, vol. 130, cols. 776–777, 15 February 1944.

21 Arthur Marwick, 'Introduction,' in *Total War and Social Change*, ed. Arthur Marwick (London: Palgrave, 1988), xvi.

22 Paul Addison, *The Road to 1945: British Politics and the Second World War* (London: Quartet, [1975] 1977), 14.

the British public and its politicians were, in fact, far from united in a desire to build and maintain this New Jerusalem and historians have long debated the extent to which there was a consensus.[23] As Ben Pimlott argues, 'Like most historical theories, the consensus thesis is as much about the present as the past. The assumption of harmony in the past is a way of underlining the gulf that is believed to exist in the present.'[24]

In 2020, when Britain was once again facing a threat and impositions like no other, the press and politicians immediately turned to these myths of Second World War to describe this new crisis in easily understood, familiar terms. How then have these myths shaped the discourse surrounding the Covid-19 crisis and to what effect?

Covid-19, The Second World War and British Political Culture

As noted above, the *Sunday Times*, in reporting on the imposition of lockdown measures in March 2020 drew heavily upon the Second World War to illustrate its point.

> The last time the British state began a multiple service attack on a lurking enemy – D-Day in 1944 – it became known as The Longest Day. On Thursday one cabinet minister reflected: 'It feels like the longest week. It felt like Brexit was going to change the country but it is the coronavirus that will do that now.'[25]

Importantly here, the *Sunday Times*, were clearly taking the cue from the unnamed cabinet minister alluding to D-Day, in describing the imposition of lockdown as the 'longest week'. The *Sunday Times* were hardly the first or last to present the crisis as akin to a war – a comparison which has elicited much criticism from historians.[26] Indeed, the Prime Minister himself had, in the days prior,

---

23 For a brief summary of the consensus debate, see: Brian Harrison, 'The Rise, Fall And Rise Of Political Consensus In Britain Since 1940,' *History* 84:274 (1999), 302–308.

24 Ben Pimlott, 'The Myth of Consensus,' in *The Making of Britain: Echoes of Greatness*, ed. Lesley M. Smith (London: Macmillan Education Ltd., 1988), 135.

25 Shipman, Wheeler, 'Ten days that shook Britain,' *Sunday Times*, 22 March 2020, 6,.

26 Arne Kislenko, 'Comparing COVID-19 To Past World War Efforts Is Premature — And Presumptuous,' *The Conversation*, 12 July 2020, https://theconversation.com/comparing-covid-19-to-past-world-war-efforts-is-premature-and-presumptuous-140701, accessed 24 May 2021; Henry Irving, *et al.*, 'The Real Lessons Of The Blitz For Covid-19,' *History & Policy*, 3 April 2020, http://www.historyandpolicy.org/policy-papers/papers/the-real-lessons-of-the-blitz-for-covid-19, accessed 24 May 2021; Martin Gorsky, 'Is

announced that 'we must act like any wartime government and do whatever it takes to support our economy' and defeat the coronavirus 'enemy'. By extension, if he was now at the head of a "wartime government" then he was a "wartime Prime Minister".[27] Notably, Johnson was far from unique in deploying this strategy. Across the Atlantic Ocean, President Donald Trump similarly attempted to position himself as a 'wartime president'.[28]

On the one hand, clearly Johnson, who had previously written a biography of Churchill[29] (a thinly veiled literary audition for his political hero's former job in No. 10 Downing Street), had positioned himself as the new 'man of destiny' for the Covid-19 crisis. In this characterisation, elements of the largely right-wing British print media were keen to assist. When Johnson was himself struck down with Covid-19, the columnist Allison Pearson took to the pages of the *Daily Telegraph*, to claim that Johnson was elevated to a 'rambunctious hero', brutally victimised by a virus laying 'siege to the country, suspending the life and liberty that no one values more than he does'. Indeed, Johnson had come, in Pearson's view, to embody the nation and its struggle against the virus itself. She concluded, 'His health is our health; if he can defeat coronavirus, then so can we. During this crucial chapter in our history, we need the narrator of our national story as never before.'[30]

Yet, given the scale of the problem, which posed massive logistical problems in terms of the provision of healthcare and rolling out a functional test and trace system, as well as cooperation from the pubic as a whole to engage with lockdown, the 'war' against Covid-19 was also to be a 'People's War'. This was a point not lost on Johnson. On 23 March 2020 he addressed the nation stating that 'in this fight we

---

COVID-19 a Crisis Like World War Two? Not Really,' *London School of Hygiene and Tropical Medicine*, 9 April 2020, https://www.lshtm.ac.uk/newsevents/expert-opinion/covid-19-crisis-world-war-two-not-re ally, accessed 24 May 2021; Richard Overy, 'Why The Cruel Myth Of The 'Blitz Spirit' Is No Model For How To Fight Coronavirus,' *Guardian*, 19 March 2020, https://www.theguardian.com/commentisfree/ 2020/mar/19/myth-blitz-spirit-model-coronavirus, accessed 21 May 2021.
27 Boris Johnson, 'Speech: Prime Minister's Statement on Coronavirus (COVID-19),' 17 March 2020, https://www.gov.uk/government/speeches/pm-statement-on-coronavirus-17-march-2020, accessed 24 May 2021.
28 Caitlin Oprysko, 'Trump Labels Himself "A Wartime President" Combating Coronavirus,' *Politico*, 18 March 2020, https://www.politico.com/news/2020/03/18/trump-administration-self-swab-co ronavirus-tests-135590, accessed 24 May 2021.
29 Boris Johnson, *The Churchill Factor: How One Man Made History* (London: Hodder & Stroughton, 2014).
30 Allison Pearson, 'Only Now Do We Realise How Valuable Boris is to Us All," *The Daily Telegraph*, 8 April 2020, 20.

can be in no doubt that each and every one of us is directly enlisted. Each and every one of us is now obliged to join together.'[31] Though clearly keen to present himself as a Churchillian figure, the 'man of destiny' for the times, it was also important to position the response of his government as leading a united Britain. Similarly, a wartime government eventually required a 'post-war' vision, which directly alluded to and incorporated the left-wing mythologies of Britain's Second World War. To this end, in a speech given in October 2020, pitching his tent firmly in the Labour Party's historical territory, he proclaimed that: 'In the depths of the second world war, in 1942 when just about everything had gone wrong, the government sketched out a vision of the post war new Jerusalem that they wanted to build. And that is what we are doing now – in the teeth of this pandemic.'[32]

This 'People's War' view of the Covid-19 crisis, was also one plainly shared by the press and other elements of Britain's political ecosystem. The *Financial Times*, for instance, quoted the Secretary of State for Health, Matt Hancock, who was even more explicit in invoking the People's War than his Prime Minister: "Our generation has never been tested like this. Our grandparents were, during the second world war, when our cities were bombed during the Blitz. Despite the pounding every night, the rationing, the loss of life, they pulled together in one gigantic national effort."[33] This, Jonathan Ford, also of the *Financial Times*, plainly agreed with, writing that Britain, 'With its memories of communal sacrifice leading to ultimate triumph, the second world war looms large in Britain's national consciousness.' But with the caveat that 'the "mobilisation" required to beat coronavirus may have a different shape and rhythm from those distant events.'[34]

Clearly then, at least three myths of the Second World War were key to both explaining and making palatable the Covid-19 crisis and its' incumbent restrictions to the British public. As a touchpoint, the war provided an important refer-

---

31 Boris Johnson, 'Speech: Prime Minister's Statement on Coronavirus (COVID-19)', 23 March 2020, https://www.gov.uk/government/speeches/pm-address-to-the-nation-on-coronavirus-23-march-2020, accessed 13 May 2022.

32 Boris Johnson, 'The Prime Minister's Full Text. He Says That, Like Churchill's Wartime Government, He Is Sketching Out A Vision Of A New Jerusalem,' *Conservative Home*, 6 October 2020, https://www.conservativehome.com/parliament/2020/10/the-prime-ministers-full-text-he-says-that-like-churchills-wartime-government-his-is-sketching-out-a-vision-of-a-new-jerusalem.html, accessed 23 February 2021.

33 Laura Hughes, 'UK To Ask Over-70s To Self-Isolate For Up To Four Months,' *Financial Times*, 15 March 2020, https://www.ft.com/content/26cc9170-669f-11ea-800d-da70cff6e4d3, accessed 24 May 2021.

34 Jonathan Ford, 'The New Wartime Economy In The Era Of Coronavirus,' *Financial Times*, 25 March 2020, https://www.ft.com/content/5945c61a-6dc7-11ea-89df-41bea055720b, accessed 24 May 2021.

ence point indicating the scale or the problem, the type of invasive response which the government would employ, and as a source of favourable, populist political rhetoric with which to couch that response. These myths were the 'man of destiny', as embodied first by Churchill and then 80 years later, by Boris Johnson. Second, the 'People's War', the myth that the British people were unified by a single cause: the defeat of the Axis powers. In 2020, that enemy had been replaced by the novel SARS-CoV-2 virus. Third, the myth of a New Jerusalem, that the extraordinary and invasive economic measures of wartime led inexorably to a new Britain, where the newly empowered Labour government of 1945, having learned the lessons of the Second World War, went on to enact its radical, egalitarian vision of the post-war society. In 2020, the same arguments were seized upon by Conservative Party Ministers to justify their own economic policies during Covid-19.

#RecordCovid19

Interestingly, though plainly hugely significant tools in framing the Covid-19 crisis, the *#RecordCovid19* project shows surprisingly little evidence that these narratives and myths from the Second World War, applied to the pandemic, cut through to the public – or at least that small section of the public who submitted their experiences to the project.

The first observation to note is that of the 119 'diary' entries submitted to the project, some 76 emerged from individuals who explicitly listed their location as being in the United Kingdom. Of those entries, only five directly discuss the war.[35] The diarist most concerned by the war in terms of the volume of her commentary on it, diarist 17, is a sales representative, a grandmother from the Northwest of the United Kingdom, aged 57. In her entry, she compared the experience of lockdown and, more explicitly, demonstrated a stoicism regarding becoming acclimatised to fear and panic prompted by the situation.

---

35 [*#RecordCovid19*–3] Lincoln, Stage manager, Female, 29 http://kristopherlovell.com/2020/04/12/record-covid-19-3-lincoln-stage-manager-female-29/, accessed 14 April 2023; [*#RecordCovid19*–17] North West UK, Sales Rep, Female 57 yrs old http://kristopherlovell.com/2020/04/22/record-covid-19-17north-west-uk-sales-rep-female-57-yrs-old/, accessed 14 April 2023; [*#RecordCovid19*–43, Student, Female, 20 http://kristopherlovell.com/2020/05/01/record-covid19-43-student-female-20/, accessed 14 April 2023; [*#RecordCovid19*–51] Suffolk, England, Postgrad Student, Female, 22, http://kristopherlovell.com/2020/05/11/recordcovid19-51-suffolk-england-postgrad-student-female-22/, accessed 14 April 2023; [*#RecordCovid19*–84] London, Office Worker, Female, 40 something, http://kristopherlovell.com/2020/10/05/recordcovid19-84-london-office-worker-female-40-something/, accessed 14 April 2023.

I often wondered how folk coped when living through the war years, the prospect of being bombed etc. I sort of get it now. Corona virus is a deadly threat –but it's impossible to keep at that high level of intense panic all the time. I find that when looking at the national figure of deaths . . . . I couldn't take it in. A couple of the earlier totals added to over 900 in a couple of days.[36]

As Penny Summerfield has shown, in her study of women's wartime memories collected through oral history interviews, some women reflected on and presented their own experiences of war as an act of 'stoic coping', which were compared sometimes unfavourably to the heroism of those in active military service.[37]

Diarist 17, continuing the allusion to the Second World War, compared front-line NHS workers to soldiers. The entry was submitted on 22 April 2020. By that stage of the pandemic at least 21,045 people in Britain had died,[38] contact tracing was in its infancy and subject to severe structural shortcomings,[39] and the NHS stockpiles of ventilators and Personal Protective Equipment (PPE) were running dangerously low.[40] These failures were keenly felt by diarist 17 who wrote:

We have one of the worst death tolls in the world. Why? Questions need to be asked and answered and people held to account. We owe it to all the families that have lost loved ones and to the NHS and other staff, killed 'in the line of duty'. It has been described frequently as a war . . . and staff 'on the front line'. However, the soldiers in this war didn't know it was coming, are amongst the lowest paid and have gone into battle without proper protective equipment.[41]

As Summerfield observed of one of her interviewees in the Second World War, the interviewee stoically survived the humdrum of wartime while her military serviceman father was a hero. In this instance, diarist 17 presents herself as stoically surviving Covid-19, increasingly numbed to the scale of death and restriction. The heroes, the health workers, were however being badly let down by an incompetent government.

---

36 [*#RecordCovid19*-17] North West UK, Sales Rep, Female 57 yrs old, http://kristopherlovell.com/ 2020/04/22/record-covid-19-17north-west-uk-sales-rep-female-57-yrs–old/, accessed 14 April 2023.

37 Penny Summerfield, 'Oral History as an Autobiographical Practice,' *Miranda* 12 (2016), https:// doi.org/10.4000/miranda.8714. For a wider discussion see also: Penny Summerfield, *Reconstructing Women's Wartime Lives* (Manchester: Manchester University Press, 1997).

38 Worldometer, 2021, 'United Kingdom Coronavirus Cases,' https://www.worldometers.info/coro navirus/uk/, accessed 25 May 2021.

39 Jonathan Calvert and George Arbuthnott, *Failures of State: The Inside Story of Britain's Battle with Coronavirus* (London: Mudlark, 2021), 98–100.

40 *BBC News*, 'Coronavirus: UK Failed to Stockpile Crucial PPE,' 28 April 2020, https://www.bbc. co.uk/news/newsbeat-52440641, accessed 25 May 2021.

41 [*#RecordCovid19*–17] North West UK, Sales Rep, Female 57 yrs old, http://kristopherlovell.com/ 2020/04/22/record-covid-19-17north-west-uk-sales-rep-female-57-yrs-old/, accessed 14 April 2023.

Another respondent to reflect on the analogies of wartime is diarist 43, a female, history student, aged 20. As a history student, diarist 43 noted that 'the reality at home is that all of us are healthy, positive and carrying on – something I reflect on as a little reminiscent of attitudes such as the blitz spirit (although of course, in a very different context).' Interestingly, Johnson and the government's efforts to present themselves as wartime leaders, appeared to hit home.

> This is another prospect I find interesting as a history student. I don't think I ever understood the rather deep relationship between a Prime Minister and the state of public attitude during war, or times of great strain. I honestly never thought I'd be waiting each day to see a figure like Boris Johnson or Dominic Raab [Secretary of State for Foreign, Commonwealth and Development Affairs] speak at a podium, and yet here I am.[42]

By contrast, diarist 3, a female Stage Manager aged 29, compared Johnson unfavourably to Churchill. In particular, as a theatrical arts professional, she worried that the government's financial support system for the self-employed would be insufficient and negatively impact her industry. As a result of this perceived failure she concluded, 'I have often heard that during WW2 Winston Churchill was told to cut funding to the arts to fund the war effort, and his reply was "Then what are we fighting for?" The same still applies today.'[43]

Diarist 51, a female postgraduate student aged 22, also noted the efforts in by the media and government to place the Covid-19 crisis within the context of British cultural memories of the Second World War. However, the wartime references did not have the desired effect. In fact, the reverse was the case, the diarist viewing such patriotic displays as a distraction from the perceived incompetence of Johnson's government.

> I feel like I'm in the incinerator from Toy Story 3, trying desperately to run from a massive fiery hole, and someone's at the controls, and everyone's screaming for them to do something and they're just singing Vera Bloody Lynn as though if we were all a little more gung-ho and Blitz Spirited about this then we'd all be muddling along nicely. I hate that our country is nearly the laughing stock of the world. I hate the idea that smug people are going to be blaming us for Boris Johnson.[44]

---

42 [*#RecordCovid19*-43] Student, Female, 20, http://kristopherlovell.com/2020/05/01/record-covid19-43-student-female-20/, accessed 14 April 2023.

43 [*#RecordCovid19*-3] Lincoln, Stage Manager, Female, 29, http://kristopherlovell.com/2020/04/12/record-covid-19-3-lincoln-stage-manager-female-29/, accessed 14 April 2023.

44 [*#RecordCovid19*-51] Suffolk, England, Postgrad Student, Female, 22, http://kristopherlovell.com/2020/05/11/recordcovid19-51-suffolk-england-postgrad-student-female-22/, accessed 14 April 2023.

Finally, diarist 84, briefly alluded to the war and, interestingly to the memory of the war. A female office worker in her 40s, she wondered whether individuals would continue to discuss their own experiences of the Covid-19 pandemic after the event concludes. The argument being that while the Second World War looms large in popular culture, individual memories of trauma and loss from that period did not. 'Everyone mentioned "the war"', the diarist believes, 'but no one wanted to talk about their individual experiences of it – because everyone who had been through it felt the same.' As such, bitter and painful memories were not passed down to those who did not live through the war years. In the case of Covid-19, the view of the diarist is that 'Everyone just wants to put it in a box, draw a line under it. Because everyone has shared it there is no need to try and explain it, as with a unique and individual trauma.'[45] The result being that, as with the Second World War, popular culture will remain, but individual experience of the trauma of the pandemic will fade.

Clearly, then, the *#RecordCovid19* project suggests that some of the wartime messaging did have an impact on a small number of the diarists, but that this was as likely to produce a negative reaction (at least among this self-selecting sample) as a positive one. In general, however, diarists overwhelmingly did not comment on the Second World War at all. In fact, just 7% of entries (submitted at the time of writing) made any reference to the conflict. Instead, diarists were far more concerned with narrating the impact of the extraordinary measures imposed by the government on their own lives and those of their families and friends. In addition, a theme running throughout the entries was the perceived risk of death or illness, again reflecting the risks to themselves and loved ones.

Of course, *#RecordCovid19* is a self-selecting qualitative collection of diaries. As noted, 76 of the diarists reported that they are from the United Kingdom, yet clearly fifteen of the entries were produced by individuals who had already contributed to the project. As such there are 61 entries by unique individuals. 34 (56%) of 61 of the diarists reported that they are female, 17 (28%) that they were male, three (5%) that they are non-binary and seven (11%) gave no response. 48 (79%) of the respondents that they are under the age of 35, 7 (11%) that they were over the age of 35, and six (10%) either did not give an age or placed themselves within a wide range. Further there were 23 students (38%), six teachers or trainee teachers (10%). The rest are spread over a range of largely professional or service industry occupations such as the civil service, administration, sales or unemployed. Clearly then, the diaries are largely submitted by younger people and

---

45 [*#RecordCovid19*-84] London, Office Worker, Female, 40 Something, http://kristopherlovell.com/2020/10/05/recordcovid19-84-london-office-worker-female-40–something/, accessed 14 April 2023.

predominantly women, thus are not reflective of wider British society. The sample provided also is clearly slanted towards the educated, many of the contributors being students or in professional occupations. Indeed, 15 of the diarists, some 25% of the sample, are female students in their late teens or early 20s. If the sample is not representative of the wider British public, it might however be representative of a largely educated, younger and predominantly female demographic.

Conclusion

It is clear that the myths, memories and cultural legacies of the Second World War have played a profound role in reactions to the Covid-19 crisis of 2020 and 2021. Like the Second World War, the pandemic has required massive effort by the state and public alike to overcome the extraordinary challenges posed by the crisis. During the Second World War, state intervention led to conscription, the direction of labour and industry, the evacuation of the cities of children and pregnant women, and massive economic controls among many other interventions by the government. During the Covid-19 crisis, the government has again been required to step in, restrict the movement of citizens, require the donning of face masks in public spaces and the effective suspension of vast swathes of the economy. This has been combined with a massive effort to procure PPE, vaccines and other health related products. In order to explain and encourage the public to engage with restrictions, unsurprisingly the government turned to the ingrained memory of the Second World War. The press and other media outlets dutifully followed suit and the key myths of the war have loomed large in discourse regarding the Covid-19 crisis.

Cultural historians of Britain's Second World War have been convinced that the role and place of the conflict in British cultural memory has little sign of diminishing. Geoff Eley went as far as to suggest that a person need not have lived through the second world war to have an ingrained memory of it, so ubiquitous is it in cultural memory.[46] Surprisingly, given the status of the war in British culture and the efforts by the state and Britain's media organs to link the crisis to that past, very few diarists – primarily younger people under the age of 35 and women – in the *#RecordCovid19* Project reflected on the war at all. Only five individuals commented in their diaries on the Second World War, despite the emphasis upon comparing the Covid-19 crisis to the war by both politicians, the print

---

46 Geoff Eley, 'Foreword,' in *British Cultural Memory and the Second World War*, eds. Lucy Noakes and Juliette Pattinson (London: Bloomsbury, 2014), xi–xxi.

media and other commentators. Indeed, one of the five diarists who did draw the comparison was aged 57 and another a history student at university – individuals perhaps more likely to be attuned, based on age and education, to such historical comparison. This may suggest that evoking an increasingly distant war, not of their parents or even grandparents' generation, has produced only limited return with the generation largely sampled. This might reflect a rejection of the comparison, alternatively it may suggest that the war is increasingly less relevant among the current generation of young, educated adults.

References

Addison, Paul. *The Road to 1945: British Politics and the Second World War.* London: Quartet, [1975] 1977.

BBC News. "Coronavirus: UK failed to stockpile crucial PPE." 28 April 2020. https://www.bbc.co.uk/news/newsbeat-52440641. Accessed 25 May 2021.

Barthes, Roland. 'Myth Today.' In *Mythologies,* edited by Roland Barthes, translated by Annette Lavers. London: Vintage, [1957] 2009.

Beveridge, William. *Social Insurance and Allied Services: Report by Sir William Beveridge.* London: HMSO, 1942.

Calder, Angus. *The Myth of the Blitz.* London: Cape, 1991.

Calder, Angus. *The People's War: Britain, 1939–1945.* London: Pimlico, 1969.

Calvert, Jonathan, and George Arbuthnott. *Failures of State: The Inside Story of Britain's Battle with Coronavirus.* London: Mudlark, 2021.

Connelly, Mark. *We Can Take It: Britain and the Memory of the Second World War.* Harlow: Pearson, 2004.

Coster, Howard. "Bird, (Cyril) Kenneth [Fougasse] (1887–1965)." *Oxford Dictionary of National Biography.* Oxford: Oxford University Press, 2004. https://www.oxforddnb.com/view/10.1093/ref:odnb/9780198614128.001.0001/odnb-9780198614128-e-1002870. Accessed 24 May 2021.

Eley, Geoff. 'Foreword' In *British Cultural Memory and the Second World War,* edited by Lucy Noakes and Juliette Pattinson, xi-xxi. London: Bloomsbury, 2014.

Gorsky, Martin. 'Is COVID-19 a Crisis Like World War Two? Not Really.' London School of Hygiene and Tropical Medicine, 9 April 2020. https://www.lshtm.ac.uk/newsevents/expert-opinion/covid-19-crisis-world-war-two-not-really. Accessed 24 May 2021.

Irving, Henry., Rosemary Cresswell, Barry Doyle, Shane Ewen, Mark Roodhouse, Charlotte Tomlinson and Marc Wiggam. 'The real lessons of the Blitz for Covid-19." *History & Policy,* 3 April 2020. http://www.historyandpolicy.org/policy-papers/papers/the-real-lessons-of-the-blitz-for-covid-19. Accessed 24 May 2021.

Ford, Jonathan. 'The New Wartime Economy In The Era Of Coronavirus.' *Financial Times,* 25 March 2020. https://www.ft.com/content/5945c61a-6dc7-11ea-89df-41bea055720b. Accessed 24 May 2021.

Fielding, Steven., Bill Schwartz and Richard Toye. *The Churchill Myths.* Oxford: Oxford University Press, 2020.

Harrison, Brian. 'The Rise, Fall And Rise Of Political Consensus In Britain Since 1940'. *History* 84:274 (1999): 302–308.

Herneman, Russel., Julian Osbaldstone, and Tony Bell. "Careless Walk Costs Lives." *The Times.* 22 March 2020. https://www.thetimes.co.uk/article/coronavirus-ten-days-that-shook-britain-and-changed-the-nation-for-ever-spz6sc9vb. Accessed 24 May 2021.

Hughes, Laura. 'UK To Ask Over-70s To Self-Isolate For Up To Four Month.' *Financial Times,* 15 March 2020. https://www.ft.com/content/26cc9170-669f-11ea-800d-da70cff6e4d3. Accessed 24 May 2021.

Johnson, Boris. "Prime Minister's Letter To Nation On Coronavirus." UK Government, 28 March 2020. https://www.gov.uk/government/publications/pm-letter-to-nation-on-coronavirus. Accessed May 24, 2021.

Johnson, Boris. "Prime Minister's Statement On Coronavirus (COVID-19)." UK Government, 17 March 2020. https://www.gov.uk/government/speeches/pm-statement-on-coronavirus-17-march-2020. Accessed 24 May 2021.

Johnson, Boris. "Prime Minister's statement on coronavirus (COVID-19)." UK Government, 23 March 2020. https://www.gov.uk/government/speeches/pm-address-to-the-nation-on-coronavirus-23-march-2020. Accessed 13 May 2022.

Johnson, Boris. *The Churchill factor: How One Man Made History.* London: Hodder & Stroughton, 2014.

Johnson, Boris. "The Prime Minister's Full Text. He Says That, Like Churchill's Wartime Government, He Is Sketching Out A Vision Of A New Jerusalem." *Conservative Home,* 6 October 2020. https://www.conservativehome.com/parliament/2020/10/the-prime-ministers-full-text-he-says-that-like-churchills-wartime-government-his-is-sketching-out-a-vision-of-a-new-jerusalem.html. Accessed 23 February 2021.

Kislenko, Arne. 'Comparing COVID-19 To Past World War Efforts Is Premature – And Presumptuous.' *The Conversation,* 12 July 2020. https://theconversation.com/comparing-covid-19-to-past-world-war-efforts-is-premature-and-presumptuous-140701. Accessed 24 May 2021.

Lovell, Kristopher. *#RecordCovid19 Project,* https://kristopherlovell.com/category/recordcovid19-project/. Accessed 14 April 2023.

Marwick, Arthur. 'Introduction'. In *Total War and Social Change,* edited by Arthur Marwick, i-xxi. London: Palgrave, 1988.

Noakes, Lucy and Juliette Pattinson. 'Introduction: 'Keep Calm and Carry On': The cultural memory of the Second World War in Britain." In *British Cultural Memory and the Second World War,* edited by Lucy Noakes and Juliette Pattinson, 1–24. London: Bloomsbury, 2014.

Oprysko, Caitlin. 'Trump Labels Himself "A Wartime President" Combating Coronavirus.' *Politico,* 18 March 2020. https://www.politico.com/news/2020/03/18/trump-administration-self-swab-coronavirus-tests-135590. Accessed 24 May 2021.

Overy, Richard. 'Why The Cruel Myth Of The "Blitz Spirit" is No Model For How To Fight Coronavirus.' *Guardian,* 19 March 2020. https://www.theguardian.com/commentisfree/2020/mar/19/myth-blitz-spirit-model-coronavirus. Accessed May 21, 2021.

Pearson, Alison. 'Only Now Do We Realise How Valuable Boris is To Us All.' *The Daily Telegraph,* April 8, 2020.

Pimlott, Ben. 'The Myth of Consensus.' In *The Making of Britain: Echoes of Greatness,* edited by Lesley M. Smith, 129–142. London: Macmillan Education Ltd. 1999.

Rose, Sonya O. *Which People's War?: National Identity and Citizenship in Wartime Britain 1939–1945* (Oxford: Oxford University Press, 2003).

Rousso, Henry. *The Vichy Syndrome: History and Memory in France since 1944.* Translated by Arthur Goldhammer. Cambridge, MA: Harvard University Press, [1987] 1991.

Shipman, Tim, and Caroline Wheeler. 'Ten Days That Shook Britain – And Changed The Nation For Ever; The Inside Story Of How Boris Johnson Changed His Priorities: Save Lives First, And Then Salvage The Economy.' *The Sunday Times*, 22 March 2020.

Smith, Alexander. 'Britain's Covid Daily Death Toll Is One Of The Worst In The World. What Went Wrong?' *NBC News*, 22 January 2021. https://www.nbcnews.com/news/world/britain-s-covid-daily-death-toll-one-worst-world-what-n1255261. Accessed 24 May 2021.

Smith, Malcolm. *Britain And 1940: History, Myth And Popular Memory*. London: Routledge, 2000.

Stevenson, John. "The New Jerusalem." In *The Making of Britain: Echoes of Greatness*, edited by Lesley M. Smith, 53–70. London: Macmillan Education Ltd. 1988.

Summerfield, Penny. 'Oral History as an Autobiographical Practice.' *Miranda*, 12 (2016). http://dx.doi.org/10.4000/miranda.8714.

Summerfield, Penny. *Reconstructing Women's Wartime Lives*. Manchester, Manchester University Press, 1997.

Summerfield, Penny. 'Women, War and Social Change: Women in Britain in World War II.' In *Total War and Social Change*, edited by Arthur Marwick, 95–118. London: Palgrave, 1988.

COVID-19 Excess Mortality Collaborators. 'Estimating Excess Mortality Due To The COVID-19 Pandemic: A Systematic Analysis Of COVID-19-Related Mortality, 2020–21.' *Lancet* 399:10334 (2022): 1513–1536. https://doi.org/10.1016/S0140-6736(21)02796-3.

Worldometer. "Coronavirus Statistics." https://www.worldometers.info/coronavirus/. Accessed 13 May 2022.

Franziska E. Kohlt
Chapter Six
A 'War' Against a 'Devilish' Virus: Religious Rhetoric and Covid-19 in the UK

Introduction: Covid 'Saints' and 'Devilish' Virus

At the start of 2021, one year into the Covid-19 pandemic, the illness and death of Sir Thomas "Captain Tom" Moore elicited an extraordinary outpouring of national grief, which captured a peculiar, yet characteristic feature of the UK's pandemic rhetoric culture. Moore, an army veteran who had become the centre of public attention for raising funds for the UK's National Health Service by walking a hundred laps in the backyard of his care home, was lauded by the BBC and many other news outlets as a 'hero', a 'National Inspiration', who 'gave the Nation hope'.[1] However, media and the UK public went further, and frequently referred to him as a 'saint', while some even called for his actual canonisation, or a cultural recognition of Moore as the 'patron saint of the NHS' – a request seemingly granted a year on, when 'Captain Tom Day' was introduced to honour the elderly in society.[2]

While for a pandemic to beget a national saint would be noteworthy enough, Moore was not the only 'Covid-saint'. Individuals, like the UK's scientific advisor, Chris Whitty were rhetorically canonised, being referred to as "saints" to highlight certain qualities and actions as desirable in relation to the pandemic. But historical saints also resurfaced, with parallels being drawn between certain aspects of their historical contexts to highlight apparently similar circumstances in the pandemic present. Luxembourg's lockdown critics, for instance, united under the icon of St. Willibrord,[3] whom they co-opted as a symbol of their movement – a function he had already served in various times of national hardship and

---

1 Anon., 'Captain Sir Tom Moore: "National Inspiration" Dies With Covid-19,' BBC, 2 February 2021 https://www.bbc.co.uk/news/uk-england-beds-bucks-herts-55881753, accessed 14 April 2023.
2 Anon., 'Obituary: Captain Sir Tom Moore, a Hero Who Gave a Nation Hope,' BBC, 2 February 2021 https://www.bbc.co.uk/news/uk-52726188, accessed 14 April 2023; Anon., 'Captain Sir Tom Moore: Day planned to empower older people,' BBC, 8 December 2021, https://www.bbc.co.uk/news/uk-england-beds-bucks-herts–59564628, accessed 14 April 2023.
3 Michel Summer, 'Willibrord as a Political Actor Between Early Medieval Ireland, Britain and Merovingian Francia (658–739),' (PHD Thesis, Trinity College Dublin, 2021) https://mittelalter.hypotheses.org/26492, accessed 14 April 2023.

https://doi.org/10.1515/9783110731002-007

occupation, with whose plights lockdown had thus become rhetorically equated. From Aachen, Germany, the portentous "rediscovery" of 'St Corona', alleged 'patron saint of pandemics', and her relics, ironically perhaps in the circumstances, went viral.

The proliferation of such "Covid-saints" highlights a little-noted but pervasive phenomenon of implicit religious narrative framings of the pandemic in mainstream, often secular discourse. While the unlikely shared roles of a medieval Syrian saint and a British war veteran thus illuminate the deliberate and synthetic character of such conceptual linguistic framings, their enthusiastic reception by media and public, and the relatively little critical attention directed towards them in scholarship, highlights the urgent necessity of closer analysis of their often undermining and even damaging dynamics in science communication.

As counter-intuitively as common pandemic slogans such as "following the science" make it sound, it is *narratives* – not 'pure' scientific *fact* – which ordinarily convey, and thus interpret, medical and scientific realities for us. As Ron Curtis has noted, narratives are also so readily applied by ourselves and others that we do not *see* the narratives, but we do instead see *through* them.[4] The abundance of religious narrative, has been scrutinized in some scientific contexts, for instance in AI and environment,[5] but is routinely little-noted and thus relatively under-discussed in others, often due to their perceived counter-intuitive presence in scientific discourse, promoted by, amongst others, a persistent, yet ahistoric, assumptions about a science-religion "conflict" or separation.[6]

The enthusiastic and "viral" uptake of, for instance, such hagiographic narratives – which turn individual actors within the pandemic into saints – raises questions about the narrative power – assumed and actual – of theological framings in assumedly secular context of science. For what reasons are they so often chosen, and why do they resonate? Is there a measurable effect of these narratives, positive or negative, and does it let us measure if they live up to the expectations we have towards them? Might they, however, in fact distort realities, and could they thus have an adverse effect? Where, in relation to historic precedent, do

---

4 Ron Curtis, 'Narrative Form and Normative Force: Baconian Story-Telling in Popular Science,' *Social Studies of Science* 24:3 (1994): 419–461.

5 Beth Singler, '"Blessed by the Algorithm": Theistic Conceptions Of Artificial Intelligence In Online Discourse,' *AI & Soc* 35, (2020): 945–955; Anna Pigott 'Hocus pocus? Spirituality and Soil Care In Biodynamic Agriculture,' *EPE: Nature and Space*, 4:4 (2021): 1665–1686.

6 See for instance Jeff Hardin, Ronald L Numbers, and Ronald A Blazey, *The Warfare Between Science and Religion (The Idea That Wouldn't Die)* (Baltimore, MD: Johns Hopkins Press, 2018); James C. Ungureanu, *Science, Religion and the Protestant Tradition: Retracing the Origins of Conflict* (Pittsburgh PA: University of Pittsburgh Press 2019); John Hedley Brooke, *Science and Religion: Some Historical Perspectives* (Cambridge: CUP, 2018).

these recent Covid-narratives sit? Finally, what are the ethical implications of the answers to these questions in pandemic communication, and beyond it?

The saints of Covid are a case in point. Aachen Cathedral's curator was open as to the reasons for creating the story of St. Corona. Through a display of the relics, she hoped 'Saint Corona may be a source of hope in these difficult times.'[7] This reasoning aligned closely with the motivation for the use the narrative use of sainthood in a pandemic with the role through which Moore was framed in the UK. Yet the use of hagiographic narratives in medical crisis sits uncomfortably within criticism of hagiography in the history of science, and in science communication, as well as more general criticism of the UK's chosen narrative framings of the pandemic. Consistently employed in order to give orientation in a new and confusing situation, religious narratives furthermore acted specifically as moral compass, to signpost the "right" and "wrong" of pandemic discourse, promising certainty in an unfamiliar situation, a time of upset, and disorientation – but not without significant pitfalls.

While such pitfalls were observed widely, they were not considered under a common theoretical framework. This chapter therefore sets out to bridge this gap by reconstructing, and thus acknowledging and documenting, the religious narrative frameworks of the Covid-19 pandemic in the UK. It will analyse the particular dynamics of religious narratives in shaping knowledge-production and behaviours in this particular scientific and crisis scenario, and connect these insights to criticism of problematic narratives in science communication and the historiography of science. This will highlight, in particular, the often implicit nature and agency of religiously-founded rhetoric through not obviously linked narrative framings, for instance of Covid-as-warfare. In so doing, this chapter will highlight how apparently general narrative framings can acquire the status and ritualistic nature of religion through the resonance of rhetoric cues in culturally-specific settings. This will foreground the dynamics of covert religious narrative, and through them discuss the potential of inappropriate narrative framings to acquire further problematic and indeed counter-productive effects – a phenomenon which Dan Kahan has described as 'feral' narratives which exert a prolonged, and particularly hard-to-control effect in 'polluting science communication environments'.[8] Thus, this chapter will illustrate how the UK's

---

7 Anon., 'German Cathedral Dusts Off Relics Of St Corona, Patron Of Epidemics,' 25 March 2020, https://www.reuters.com/article/us-health-coronavirus-germany-saint-idUSKBN21C2PM, accessed 14 April 2023.

8 Dan M. Kahan. 'Protecting or Polluting the Science Communication Environment?: The Case of Childhood Vaccines,' in *The Oxford Handbook of the Science of Science Communication,* eds. Kathleen Hall Jamieson, Dan M. Kahan and Dietram A. Scheufele (Oxford: Oxford University Press, 2017), 422–432.

chosen rhetoric framings of Covid-19 implicitly acted *as* religion, by establishing a fixed moral framework that provoked unambiguous judgment calls in a dynamic medical situations whose complexities were incompatible with it, to reflect on the principles of good, or, indeed ethical, science communication, and why, in the knowledge of them, the known risks of chosen rhetoric register of the UK's crisis communication were embraced.

Britain's 'Good War' Against Covid-19

The narrative framing of the Covid-19 pandemic in the United Kingdom was seemingly decided in unison early on: the UK was "going to war" against the novel coronavirus. This framing was immediate and pervasive: Prime Minister Boris Johnson 'declared war on coronavirus', and his cabinet a 'wartime government'[9] at the onset of the pandemic in the UK, and Health Minister Matt Hancock continuously referred to government responses as a 'battle plan'.[10] This framing was conscious and deliberate, and patterns of its use indicate its strategic deployment. Abundant especially during the "first wave", subsequent periods of intensified war rhetoric coincided with periods of introduction and reintroduction of lockdown measures, which, as I have examined elsewhere, in turn, also corresponded to increased death rates.[11] After loosening of lockdown measures, and renewed increases in death rates, war rhetoric returned with renewed strength in September 2020, when the Health Secretary's House of Commons statement made reference to the 'common enemy' and other such terms established earlier on several times a minute.[12]

---

9 Boris Johnson, 'Prime Minister's Statement on Coronavirus (COVID-19),' 17 March 2020, https://www.gov.uk/government/speeches/pm-statement-on-coronavirus-17-march-2020, accessed 14 April 2023.
Boris Johnson, 'Prime Minister's Statement on Coronavirus (COVID-19),' 10 May 2020, https://www.gov.uk/government/speeches/pm-address-to-the-nation-on-coronavirus-10-may-2020, accessed 14 April 2023.
10 Matt Hancock, 'Health Secretary Sets Out Government "Battle Plan" For COVID-19,' 1 March 2020, https://www.gov.uk/government/news/health-secretary-sets-out-government-battle-plan-for-covid-19, accessed 14 April 2023.
11 Franziska Kohlt, "Over by Christmas": The Impact Of War-Metaphors And Other Science-Religion Narratives On Science Communication Environments During The Covid-19 Crisis.' Preprint, *SocArXiv*, November 2020, https://doi.org/10.31235/osf.io/z5s6a.
12 Matt Hancock, 'Health and Social Care Secretary's Statement On Coronavirus (COVID-19),' 28 April 2020, https://www.gov.uk/government/speeches/health-and-social-care-secretarys-statement-on-coronavirus-covid-19-28-april-2020, accessed 14 April 2023.

War-rhetoric is not, on the surface, religious narrative, it became, as this chapter will show, its prime vehicle. It is therefore, first of all, necessary to acknowledge commonalities of the usage of this rhetoric, before analysing its distinctiveness. That the war-framing was a common narrative response to Covid-19, and one notably not exclusive to the UK, was noted by numerous journalistic and academic articles.[13] France's President Emmanuel Macron had also 'declared war' on the virus early on, and New York City's mayor Andrew Cuomo would go on to say that 'Ventilators are to this war what bombs were to World War Two'.[14] Analysis of historical medical crisis communication also shows that this has been a common response historically, for instance during the HIV and Zika crises,[15] and is also, more generally, a common framing for individual illness, for instance in cancer.[16] All these analyses also unanimously agree that the use of war rhetoric in medical contexts is 'ironic, unfortunate and unnecessary'.[17]

The way in which the warfare framings of Covid-19 manifested in the UK were distinct and culturally specific in ways that made them susceptible to become the vehicle of religious narrative, which is, in turn, illustrated in their transcendence from political leadership into public use. This transition was top-down, coordinated, and immersive, spreading first via political leadership into wider circulation, and subsequently through press and broadcast media into general use. The titular head of UK government, Queen Elizabeth II, amplified the language of her government as she recalled in a rare out of the ordinary address a popular wartime song – 'We will meet again' – thus anchoring a specific war

---

13 Richard Horton, 'Offline: COVID-19 as Culture War,' *Lancet* 399:10322, (2022): 364; Francesca Panzeri, Simona Di Paola, Filippo Domaneschi, 'Does the COVID-19 War Metaphor Influence Reasoning?,' *PLOS One* 24: 3 (2021) https://doi.org/10.1371/journal.pone.0250651.
14 Adrienne Bernhard, 'Covid-19: What We Can Learn From Wartime Efforts,' BBC Future, 1 May 2020 https://www.bbc.com/future/article/20200430-covid-19-what-we-can-learn-from-war time-efforts, accessed 14 April 2023.
15 Jing-Bao Nie et al, 'Healing Without Waging War: Beyond Military Metaphors in Medicine and HIV Cure Research,' *American Journal for Bioethics* 10 (2016): 3–11, https://doi.org/10.1080/ 15265161.2016.1214305; Dan Kahan, 'Protecting or Polluting the Science Communication Environment?: The Case of Childhood Vaccines,' in *The Oxford Handbook of the Science of Science Communication*, 422–432.
16 Judy Z Segal, *Health and the Rhetoric of Medicine* (Carbondale: Southern Illinois University Press, 2008). Judy Z Segal. 'Cancer Experience and its Narration: An Accidental Study,' *Literature and Medicine* 30:2 (2012): 292–318. Per Krogh Hansen, 'Illness and Heroics: On Counter-narrative and counter-metaphor in the discourse on cancer,' *Frontiers of Narrative Studies* 4:1 (2018): 213–228.
17 Jing-Bao Nie, Adam Gilbertson, Malcolm de Roubaix, Ciara Staunton, Anton van Niekerk, Joseph D Tucker and Stuart Rennie, 'Healing Without Waging War: Beyond Military Metaphors in Medicine and HIV Cure Research,' *American Journal for Bioethics* 10 (2016): 1.

framing prominently on the front pages of newspapers across the political spectrum.[18] The phrase was subsequently projected from Piccadilly Circus's famous billboards,[19] and could soon be found sprayed onto buildings and displayed in the windows of closed businesses illustrating how it transcended from political, and journalistic realms into popular usage.

The reference to Vera Lynn's wartime song 'We'll Meet Again' is noteworthy, as it characterises the way in which the war language that was employed in the UK was not generic. This rhetoric, firstly, drew on specific phrases, narratives, practices, and set pieces that are already culturally codified to convey a certain historiography of the world wars, especially of the second world-war as a "Good War".[20] Having evolved to become a 'key aspect of British national identity' and 'popular culture', this narrative lives on in 'artefacts' and 'numerous acts of memorialization and commemoration', and rhetoric routines surrounding it are well known, generally positively received, so that they could be relied upon for participation.[21]

Thus, common references were made to slogans popularly associated with the two World Wars in Britain. When Prime Minister Boris Johnson expressed hope to 'allow a more significant return to normality from November at the earliest – possibly in time for Christmas', for instance, several headlines reported his plans under the headline 'It'll be over by Christmas':[22] he was recalling the 'Over by Christmas' slogan. Despite the latter having been challenged with regards to

---

18 Elizabeth II, The Queen's coronavirus speech transcript: "We will succeed and better days will come," *The Telegraph*, 5 April 2020, https://www.telegraph.co.uk/news/2020/04/05/queens-coro navirus-speech-full-will-succeed-better-days-will/, accessed 14 April 2023.
19 Emmet McGonagle, 'Queen's Virus Message On London's Piccadilly Lights Wins Plaudits,' *Campaign*, 9 April 2020 https://www.campaignlive.co.uk/article/queens-virus-message-londons-pic cadilly-lights-wins-plaudits/1679849, accessed 14 April 2023.
20 Kit Kowol, 'Britain's Obsession With The Second World War And The Debates That Fuel It,' *The Conversation*, 4 June 2020 https://theconversation.com/britains-obsession-with-the-second-world-war-and-the-debates-that-fuel-it-139497, accessed 14 April 2023; AJP Taylor, *The Origins of the Second World War* (London: Penguin, 1991); BBC One Show, '"We'll Meet Again" Lyrics – VE Day Singalong' (2020) https://www.bbc.co.uk/programmes/articles/5qhhFG1vNtX8swrtg9gKQlR/ we-ll-meet-again-lyrics-ve-day-singalong, accessed 14 April 2023.
21 Lucy Noakes and Juliette Pattinson, "Keep Calm And Carry On": The Cultural Memory Of The Second World War In Britain,' in *British Cultural Memory and the Second World War* eds. Lucy Noakes and Juliette Pattinson (London: Bloomsbury, 2013), 20.
22 Marina Hyde, '"Over By Christmas": Now Where Have We Heard Johnson's New Slogan Before?' *The Guardian*, 17 July 2020https://www.theguardian.com/commentisfree/2020/jul/17/christ mas-johnson-slogan-prime-minister-pmqs, accessed 14 April 2023.

its historicity[23] it has nevertheless become popularised in the historiography of World War I.[24] Such appeals to shared cultural memory, however historically challenged, accounted for the swift uptake of this narrative framing and interpretation of the Covid-19 pandemic as a war beyond the high-profile settings in which it had come into first use. It also accounted for expectable – and expected – shared behavioural responses to such language – and through it, to the pandemic, which, despite its narrative framing, remained a medical, not a military, crisis. The imminent 'VE Day' ("Victory in Europe Day") in May 2020, which took place four weeks after the peak of the first wave of Covid-19 in the UK, became the stage for street-parties and national sing-alongs of "We'll meet again", facilitated by the national broadcaster, the BBC, in "defiance" of Covid-19, despite never previously having been celebrated in this way.

The narrative of "defiance" had at this point been established for instance Elizabeth II's speech as a show of the "Blitz Spirit". Used interchangeably with the "Dunkirk Spirit", this characterised how, as a headline accompanying singer Katherine Jenkins's rendition of "We'll Meet Again" stated, the "war against Covid-19" was 'bringing the nation together.' Notably, the medical messaging dominant at the time advocated "staying at home" to save lives, isolation and social distancing. This was diametrically opposed to what 'coming together' implied, illustrating how narrative, and the communal behaviours it anticipated, were the opposite of what scientific guidance advocated.

The directions in which this public narrative led its audience, were thus known and anticipated, and perceived as desirable in communication at a time when it directly contradicted guidance communicated by the same actors. They were furthermore well rehearsed, their popularity would have been known to these communicators. As Noakes and Pattinson have noted, what was repeated in the Covid setting, were enactments of national identity and war remembrance.[25] A previous occasion, for instance, on which Jenkins had performed "We'll Meet Again" prior to Covid was an explicitly military and national one – the 75th

---

23 Stuart Halifax, '"Over by Christmas": British Popular Opinion And The Short War In 1914,' *War Studies* 1:2 (2010), 103–121.

24 As historians have pointed out, this slogan had no equivalent contemporary currency (Halifax, 2010) – the issue of historiography vs history this raises, also characterises and highlights issues, such as the discrepancies between expectations and realities of warfare rhetoric, which will be discussed as a further aspect of the "identity" aspect of war rhetoric in health crisis, and its counterproductive effects in this discourse and beyond, will be discussed below.

25 Janet Watson, 'Total War And Total Anniversary: The Material Culture Of Second World War Commemoration In Britain,' in *British Cultural Memory and the Second World War*, eds Lucy Noakes and Juliette Pattinson. London: Bloomsbury, 2013, 175–194.

anniversary of the end of the Second World War.[26] And Covid-responses that captured this framing, consistently and most successfully captured the public imagination. The website for the BBC's VE day sing-along was adorned with WW2 Spitfire-war planes and Union Jacks, and likewise transcended being a media framing only when a fundraiser for several actual Spitfire-flyovers gathered just over £123,000.[27] This was the framework in which military veteran Captain Tom would later become the ideal, the hero, the saint-figure embodying the actions and behaviours to which to aspire in the pandemic. The BBC highlighted his foremost qualities, and, thus, the foremost desirable qualities of any Briton in a pandemic: "Captain Tom" 'was Britain as it needed to see itself: selfless, patriotic and undefeated – and never taking a backward step.'[28] Narratives of nationalism and patriotism were blended with militarism and a specific historiography of the world wars to constitute the cultural response of the UK to Covid-19.

The contrast of medical advice and behaviours elicited by this framing, already highlight that they were not unproblematic. They imposed, rhetorically, national and military virtues upon a medical, a public health crisis, in their self-declared aims of bringing "hope" and "the nation together", which were re-endorsed and prioritised by government and media acknowledgment of them. The benchmark, however, of effective narrative in science communication, and good communication, in public health crisis, is their clarity – a narrative, therefore, must clarify and amplify the scientific reality to which it is applied – and the prevention and limitation of morbidity and mortality.[29] The warfare framing problematically aligned with other contemporary nationalist narratives. With the index case of Covid and "Brexit Day" coinciding on 31 January – those critical of the warfare framing could

---

26 '"We'll Meet Again" - Katherine Jenkins brings the nation together in song | VE Day 75 - BBC', BBC <https://www.youtube.com/watch?v=SKSc8BLXAJ8>.

27 The Aircraft Restoration Company (2020) The NHS Spitfire, https://www.justgiving.com/fund raising/nhsspitfire, accessed 14 April 2023.

28 Anon., 'Obituary: Captain Sir Tom Moore, A Hero Who Gave A Nation Hope,' BBC News, 2 February 2021 https://www.bbc.co.uk/news/uk-52726188, accessed 14 April 2023.

29 Julia M. Pearce, G. James Rubin, Richard Amlôt, Simon Wessely, and M. Brooke Rogers, 'Communicating Public Health Advice After a Chemical Spill: Results From National Surveys in the United Kingdom and Poland,' *Disaster Medicine and Public Health Preparedness* 7:1 (2013), 65–74, https://doi.org/10.1001/dmp.2012.56; Alison Bish, Susan Michie and Professor Lucy Yardley, 'Principles of Effective Communication. Scientific Evidence Base Review,' *Department of Health: Pandemic Preparedness* (2010) https://www.gov.uk/government/publications/review-of-the-evidence-base-underpinning-the-uk-influenza-pandemic-preparedness-strategy, accessed 14 April 2023; Franziska Kohlt, "Over by Christmas".

especially easily be dismissed as unpatriotic.[30] War narratives produced a polarised response, failing at least one of its self-declared aims (to 'bring the nation together'), and, as the next section will show, diverted attention from, and even undermined scientific and medical guidance, influencing what actions were regarded as desirable during the pandemic, and thus actual behaviours into harmful directions.

Diffusive Religion: Sacrifice, and the 'God'-given 'Freedom' from a 'Devilish Virus'

As demonstrated with the impact of the Queen's chosen slogan, warfare narratives could be expected to elicit a generally enthusiastic response, a collective and uniform set of behaviours with a high level of uptake. Their ritualistic appearance is indicative of the religious origin of this particular rhetoric, and the problematic historical entanglements of health, national identity, military and religion in the UK that complicates their use, especially in medical crisis.

This link between war and religion, between rhetoric and ritual, manifested explicitly, for instance, in Health Secretary Matt Hancock's response to the sharp increase in deaths among health workers in the following manner at the opening of the government's daily Covid briefing:

> This morning, at 11 o'clock, we paused to remember the 85 NHS colleagues and 19 social care colleagues who have lost their lives with coronavirus. [. . .] They are the nation's fallen heroes. And we will remember them.[31]

Hancock here consciously evoked the formulae of the UK's well-known National Service of Remembrance, usually celebrated in November on Remembrance Sunday. Although the 11 o'clock silence on Remembrance Day is now observed nationally, and has widely been adopted in secular settings, its origins are in religious ceremony. The annually televised and broadcast service still processes into Westminster Abbey and is led by the incumbent Bishop of London.

---

30 Dan Hodge, 'The Left's Hate Mob Can't Stand That Boris Worked Himself Into Intensive Care To Fight (Yes, Fight!) This Virus,' *The Daily Mail*, 12 April 2020 https://www.dailymail.co.uk/de bate/article-8211341/The-Lefts-hate-mob-stand-Boris-worked-intensive-care-fight-virus.html, accessed 14 April 2023.
31 Matt Hancock, 'Health And Social Care Secretary's Statement On Coronavirus (COVID-19),' 28 April 2020, https://www.gov.uk/government/speeches/health-and-social-care-secretarys-state ment-on-coronavirus-covid-19-28-april-2020, accessed 14 April 2023.

But this deliberate appropriation of a religious ritual, previously appropriated for a military context, was not the first time Hancock used language with religious origin or from explicitly religious settings. In a televised exchange with the opposition leader, the leader of the Royal College of Nursing, and then Archbishop of York, John Sentamu, in the BBC's political programme *Question Time*, he demonstrated the code-like nature of this language. Framing his demand for a more resolute response, Sentamu asked Hancock to 'command these files' (referring to his call for military support of the Covid efforts), to which the Health Secretary responded in kind, that he would 'not cease from this fight'.[32] Both phrases refer to hymns – the first to 'My Soul, There is a Country' and the second to 'And Did Those Feet in Ancient Time (Jerusalem)' – and, notably, hymns which, popularised through war remembrance, have transitioned beyond church-use into national and patriotic settings, similar to the Service of Remembrance. 'Jerusalem' traditionally concludes the 'Last Night of the Proms', and has included at such national occasions as the London Olympic Opening Ceremony in 2012.

That both instances in which Hancock used explicitly religious narrative related to health workers appeared not coincidental, as the second dominant framing of Covid-19 discourse in the UK – the theme of "sacrifice" – became the dominant narrative to frame health professionals. Another integral part of the UK's "good war" narrative, it was also one through which its complications, when used in health contexts, become most clear. Noakes and Pattinson characterise how the "sacrifice" narrative is likewise perpetuated by remembrance culture, and annually brought to public consciousness through the Remembrance ceremony. The sacrifice that is honoured is that of soldiers – with whom health workers thus become rhetorically equated in the context of Covid-19, continuing the conflation of military and medical spheres. The words of the Exhortation, ending in 'we will remember them' repurposed by Hancock, are spoken during this national celebration, to which the liturgical elements remain structurally and thematically integral. The two-minute silence, and Exhortation, are framed with hymns and traditional music which abundantly stresses the theme of soldiers' "sacrifice", comparing it to the death of Christ, as necessary for the salvation of others.

Yet the implications of this framing, which were problematic for soldiers then, indicate some of the issues of the appropriation of this narrative in medical crisis. As Michael Snape documents, the sacrifice narrative of the World Wars was strategically-deployed among lower-class soldiers, comparing their near-inevitable deaths

---

32 BBC *Question Time*, 2 April 2020, https://www.bbc.co.uk/iplayer/episode/m000gxw2/question-time-2020–02042020, accessed 14 April 2023.

to that of Christ – a notion that persists in the hymns that colour Remembrance services to this day (eg. 'Greater Love Hath No Man', 'O Valiant Heart'). Likening the deaths of soldiers to that of Christ renders them necessary for salvation-by-victory, and, as that of Christ, can and should not be hindered. This embedded the 'rhetoric of martyrdom and sacrifice' in the 'religious dimension of British patriotism' then.[33] While this was perceived distasteful by some of those framed in this way at the time, as evident in the words of the 'War Poets', such as Wilfred Owen or Siegfried Sassoon, who felt their experiences were silenced by them,[34] death is a chosen risk, and thus more accepted outcome of the professional path of a soldier – it is not for medics. An alignment of the two does not, as a narrative in science and medical discourse should do, clarify or amplify, but, in this case, instead distorts.

The juxtaposition of this historical appropriation of Christian narrative frameworks of sacrifice, for war, and for the purpose of Covid-19, constitutes an example of what historians of war and Christianity have called "Diffusive Christianity". This has been defined as a culture in which military and Christian values and narratives become first amalgamated and then aligned: one to reinforce and justify the aims of the other.[35] It is this context in which, as Roberta Bivins makes clear, the language, narratives, and indeed mythology of the National Health Service in Britain was conceived, shaped and cultivated.[36] In this context, the institution of the NHS has, in more than just popular parlance, become 'the closest thing the English people have to a religion',[37] a nation for whom, as Alec Ryrie has asserted, the Second World War has become its 'Sacred Story'.[38] The narrative framing of Covid-19 therefore functioned *as* religion, and thus promised salvation in exchange for virtue that had become defined primarily in military and patriotic terms, to which all other terms can easily appear secondary.

---

33 Michael Snape. *God and the British Soldier: Religion and the British Army in the First and Second World War* (London and New York: Routledge, 2005), 242 & 94.

34 Santanu Das, 'Reframing First World War Poetry: An Introduction,' in *The Cambridge Companion to the Poetry of the First World War,* ed. by Santanu Das (Cambridge: Cambridge University Press, 2013).

35 John Drewett, 'Diffused Christianity: Asset or Liability?' *Theology* 45 (1942) 82–92. Callum G. Brown, *The Death of Christian Britain: Understanding Secularisation 1800–2000* (London: Routledge, 2001); Snape, *God and the British Soldier.*

36 Roberta Bivins, 'Commentary: Serving The Nation, Serving The People: Echoes Of War In The Early NHS,' *Medical Humanities* 46, (2020) 154–156.

37 Nigel Lawson, *The View from No.11: Memoirs of a Tory Radical* (London: Bantam Press, 1992).

38 Alec Ryrie, 'Our Sacred Story', BBC iPlayer, 7 November 2020, https://www.bbc.co.uk/programmes/m000p60n, accessed 14 April 2023.

In the Covid-19 pandemic, such war metaphors this complicated medical communication, and even the work of medics and scientists, in a number of ways. The narrative distortion and misrepresentation of medics was lamented and protested by members of the profession, in due course. US medic Adina Wise summarises that 'militarised diction to describe doctors' sense of duty conflates and confuses the reality of our responsibilities': 'War is dangerous by definition, but danger should never be inherent in the hospital'.[39] In the UK in particular, medics specifically resisted the framing of 'heroes' and 'sacrifice', expressing no need for 'medals and flypasts' – and 'I don't even (whisper it) need Colonel Tom (*sic*)'[40] – and felt silenced in the call for appropriate protection, 'proper pay and PPE' in their work.[41] Exasperated at the inappropriateness of the framing of patriotism as a measure, one wrote 'One cannot sing Rule Britannia to a virus'.[42] UK doctors protested outside government residence No 10 Downing Street with a sign that read "Doctors not Martyrs".[43]

Imposing a narrative, the binary opposite of what medics believed and sought to communicate, undermined the authority of medical staff, on their own working conditions, as well as appropriate measures for the public, and scientific advice communicated at government level. The hagiographic, at times even apotheotic, language applied to medical staff while intuitively positive, is thus, as research in historiography of science and science communication research has shown aligned more with the rhetoric patterns of populism, than that of good science and risk communication.[44] As Mede and Schaefer observe, especially anti-science populism relies on social portrayals of infallibility of scientists, their elevation beyond the ordinary human capabilities and knowledge, in Covid-19 as in Climate

39 Adina Wise, 'The Rhetoric Of War Implies A Heedless Approach That Undermines The Practice Of Medicine,' 17 April 2020, https://blogs.scientificamerican.com/observations/military-meta phors-distort-the-reality-of-covid-19/, accessed 14 April 2023.

40 Anon., 'I'm An NHS Doctor – And I've Had Enough Of People Clapping For Me,' *The Guardian*, 21 May 2020, https://www.theguardian.com/society/2020/may/21/nhs-doctor-enough-people-clap ping, accessed 14 April 2023.

41 Rachel Clarke, 'NHS Doctor: Forget Medals And Flypasts – What We Want Is Proper Pay and PPE,' *The Guardian*, 2 May 2020, https://www.theguardian.com/society/2020/may/02/nhs-doctor-for get-medals-and-flypasts-what-we-want-is-proper-pay-and-ppe, accessed 14 April 2023.

42 Musa Okwonga, 'You Cannot Sing "Rule Britannia" to a Virus,' *Byline Times*, 19 March 2020, https://bylinetimes.com/2020/03/19/you-cannot-sing-rule-britannia-to-a-virus/, accessed 14 April 2023.

43 Liz Gerard, 'The British People Are Being Played For Fools,' *The New European*, 3 June 2020, https://www.theneweuropean.co.uk/brexit-news-uk-population-being-fooled-by-government-82552/, accessed 14 April 2023.

44 Anna Maerker, 'Hagiography and Biography: Narratives of 'Great Men of Science' in *History, Memory and Public Life: The Past in the Present*, eds. by Adam Sutcliffe and Simmon Sleight (London: Routledge, 2018); Mary Midgley. *Science as Salvation* (London: Routledge, 2018).

Change.[45] This was particularly poignant in the ideals of pandemic sainthood promoted through "Captain Tom". Called 'unchanging', 'never taking a step back', he was framed as ideal of pandemic response, unchangeability can hardly apply to medical and scientific professionals needing to be dynamic in response to ongoing research and discoveries about a novel virus. Science, contrary to popular portrayal as purveyor of "facts", is self-refining, rather than monolithic, and thus, such narrative framings discredit scientific best practice. Martyrs and sacrifices no longer speak, no longer change: rather than elevating their expertise, such rhetoric deprioritised, undermined and silenced it.

This puts into perspective Prime Minister Boris Johnson's reluctance to introduce early pandemic protective measures, despite them being advocated by scientific advisors. Likewise expressed through the language of "Diffusive Christianity", and its conflating of divine and nationalist tropes, specifically that of national freedom in his first speech on the virus, this remained the keynote of the crisis. Linking Brexit and the threat of SARS-CoV-2, Johnson emphasised that the main achievement of the UK's departure from the European Union had been 'freedom', especially 'free trade' which he asserted was 'God's diplomacy'. Any restrictions or limitations to it in response to 'new diseases such as coronavirus' were not only 'bizarre', and 'beyond rational' – they were against the 'healthy' divine order or British freedom from their necessity; the virus itself thus 'evil' and 'devilish'.[46]

Johnson evoked the wartime speech eloquence that had first established Diffusive Christianity as a response to National hardship, such as George VI's VE Day speech in which he had not only called upon his listeners to 'remember' the 'sacrifice', but to celebrate 'freedom' and 'independence' from 'tyranny' of a 'determined and cruel foe' and 'enemy', a 'victory' and 'triumph', brought to Britain by the 'Almighty God', to whose 'virtues' the British people had adhered.[47] Yet the hope, likely it may have been really felt at the end of the war in 1945, could, at the time and in the context in which Johnson summoned it, 'not work'. Rhetoric that is not 'accompanied by facts from a credible source' essential for their credibility, and long-term positive effect – as the language of medical advice – remained

---

45 Niels G. Mede and Mike S. Schäfer, 'Science-Related Populism: Conceptualizing Populist Demands Toward Science,' *Public Understanding of Science* 29:5 (2020): 473–491.
46 Boris Johnson, 'Prime Minister's Statement on Coronavirus (COVID-19)', 10 May 2020, https://www.gov.uk/government/speeches/pm-address-to-the-nation-on-coronavirus-10-may-2020, accessed 14 April 2023; Boris Johnson, 'PM Speech in Greenwich', 3 February 2020, https://www.gov.uk/government/speeches/pm-speech-in-greenwich-3-february-2020, accessed 2023.
47 George VI's VE Day broadcast (1945), https://www.royal.uk/king-george-vis-ve-day-broadcast, accessed 14 April 2023.

opposed to narrative, as facts were not available to support hope where Johnson had wished to evoke it.[48]

The very real detrimental effect misaligned narrative framings can have in public health crisis communication were illustrated when such narratives of war and sacrifice were widened to other professional groups of 'key workers': it showed the ease with which medically untenable statements could be made within this narrative framework. As teachers, in a manner identical to medical staff, expressed concerns about work safety, they were harshly criticised by the former head of their professional supervision body, Ofsted, amplified by populist parts of the British media landscape, for lack of 'willingness' to 'sacrifice' themselves in a similar way to health workers.[49] Such headlines compounded the negative effects of such rhetoric on attitudes towards this professional group, and their experiences of the pandemic.[50] They framed teachers as unpatriotic or the enemy within. Narrative had here created a framework in which it had become desirable to ask for the sacrifice of real lives, as opposed to adhering to medical advice to protect them.

Rhetoric, Ritual – Reality? Conclusion

The dominant religious narratives of Covid-19 in the UK were deliberate, distracting and detrimental. They not only misrepresented historical warfare, but distorted and obfuscated the realities of the present. As the example of teachers showed, they were inappropriate, as they (entirely contrary to the benchmark of good science communication to preserve life and health), idealised seeking out death, and rendered necessary protective measures the opposite of 'salvation', defined as 'freedom' from them, thus actively counter-acting consensus medical guidance. As this medical guidance was communicated, amongst others, by government advisors themselves, there rhetoric choices produced contradictory messaging from the same institution, undermining its credibility, rather than sustaining trust within it.

---

48 Simon Wessely and Jo Daniels, 'Why Reassuring The Public May Not Be The Best Way To End Lockdown', KCL, 9 May 2020, https://www.kcl.ac.uk/news/why-reassuring-the-public-may-not-be-the-best-way-to-end-lockdown, accessed 14 April 2023.

49 Joe Middleton, 'Teachers Should Be Prepared To 'Sacrifice Their Lives,' Says Ex-Ofsted Head,' *Independent*, 26 February 2021, https://www.independent.co.uk/news/education/covid-schools-re opening-ofsted-teachers-b1807935.html, accessed 14 April 2023.

50 Kathryn Asbury And Lisa Kim, '"Lazy, Lazy Teachers": Teachers' Perceptions Of How Their Profession Is Valued By Society, Policymakers, And The Media During COVID-19,' Epub ahead of print 20 July 2020, https://doi.org/10.31234/osf.io/65k8q.

The perceived positives of this language upon morale, only had a short-term effect, and their community-building powers proved divisive along the same fissure lines in society already marked by their use in other populist discourses. The religious dimensions of the warfare rhetoric of Covid thus deepened and complexified the detrimental effects outlined in medical communication literature of why war narratives in these contexts are ill-advised. As the damage they can do when unintended semiotic confluences are created by specific cultural contexts, they can even constitute a threat to life, through acceptance or idealising of avoidable death. The avoidance of such narrative framing in medical crisis can therefore not be a matter of preference, but must be a matter of ethics, of equal importance as the production and dissemination of medical science and advice.

References

Anon., 'Captain Sir Tom Moore: "National inspiration" dies with Covid-19.' BBC, 2 February 2021 https://www.bbc.co.uk/news/uk-england-beds-bucks-herts-55881753. Accessed 14 April 2023.

Anon., 'Obituary: Captain Sir Tom Moore, A Hero Who Gave A Nation Hope.' BBC, 2 February 2021 https://www.bbc.co.uk/news/uk-52726188, accessed 14 April 2023.

Anon., 'Captain Sir Tom Moore: Day Planned To Empower Older People.' BBC, 8 December 2021 https://www.bbc.co.uk/news/uk-england-beds-bucks-herts-59564628. Accessed 14 April 2023.

Anon., 'I'm an NHS Doctor – And I've Had Enough Of People Clapping For me.' *The Guardian*, 21 May 2020 https://www.theguardian.com/society/2020/may/21/nhs-doctor-enough-people-clapping. Accessed 14 April 2023.

Anon., 'German cathedral dusts off relics of St Corona, patron of epidemics.' 25 March 2020 https://www.reuters.com/article/us-health-coronavirus-germany-saint-idUSKBN21C2PM. Accessed 14 April 2023.

The Aircraft Restoration Company, 'The NHS Spitfire.' 2020, https://www.justgiving.com/fundraising/nhsspitfire. Accessed 14 April 2023.

Asbury, Kathryn. and Lisa Kim, '"Lazy, Lazy Teachers": Teachers' Perceptions Of How Their Profession Is Valued By Society, Policymakers, And The Media During Covid-19.' Epub ahead of print 20 July 2020. https://doi.org/10.31234/osf.io/65k8q

BBC *One Show*, '"We'll Meet Again" Lyrics – VE Day Singalong.' 2020, https://www.bbc.co.uk/programmes/articles/5qhhFG1vNtX8swrtg9gKQIR/we-ll-meet-again-lyrics-ve-day-singalong, accessed 14 April 2023.

BBC Radio Two, 'D-Day 70 Years On – Full concert.' 6 June 2014, https://www.bbc.co.uk/programmes/b042zhm5. Accessed 14 April 2023.

BBC Question Time, BBC iPlayer, 2 April 2020, https://www.bbc.co.uk/iplayer/episode/m000gxw2/question-time-2020-02042020. Accessed 14 April 2023.

Bernhard, Adrienne. 'Covid-19: What We Can Learn From Wartime Efforts.' BBC 1 May 2020, https://www.bbc.com/future/article/20200430-covid-19-what-we-can-learn-from-wartime-efforts. Accessed 14 April 2023.

Bish, Alison., Susan Michie and Lucy Yardley, 'Principles of Effective Communication. Scientific Evidence Base Review.' *Department of Health: Pandemic Preparedness*. (2010) https://www.gov. uk/government/publications/review-of-the-evidence-base-underpinning-the-uk-influenza-pandemic-preparedness-strategy. Accessed 14 April 2023.

Bivins, Roberta. 'Commentary: Serving The Nation, Serving The People: Echoes Of War In The Early NHS.' *Medical Humanities* 46, (2020): 154–156.

Brown, Callum G., *The Death of Christian Britain: Understanding Secularisation 1800–2000*. London: Routledge, 2001.

Clarke, Rachel., 'NHS Doctor: Forget Medals And Flypasts – What We Want Is Proper Pay And PPE.' *The Guardian*, 2 May 2020, https://www.theguardian.com/society/2020/may/02/nhs-doctor-forget-medals-and-flypasts-what-we-want-is-proper-pay-and-ppe. Accessed 14 April 2023.

Curtis, Ron. 'Narrative Form and Normative Force: Baconian Story-Telling in Popular Science.' *Social Studies of Science*. 24:3 (1994): 419–461.

Das, Santanu. 'Reframing First World War Poetry: An Introduction.' In *The Cambridge Companion to the Poetry of the First World War*, edited by Santanu Das. Cambridge: Cambridge University Press, 2013.

Drewett John. 'Diffused Christianity: Asset or Liability?' *Theology* 45 (1942): 82–92.

George VI's VE Day broadcast (1945). https://www.royal.uk/king-george-vis-ve-day-broadcast, accessed 14 April 2023.

Elizabeth II, The Queen's coronavirus speech transcript: "We Will Succeed And Better Days Will Come." *The Telegraph*, 5 April 2020 https://www.telegraph.co.uk/news/2020/04/05/queens-coronavirus-speech-full-will-succeed-better-days-will/. Accessed 14 April 2023.

Gerard, Liz. 'The British People Are Being Played For Fools.' *The New European*, 3 June 2020. https://www.theneweuropean.co.uk/brexit-news-uk-population-being-fooled-by-government-82552/. Accessed 14 April 2023.

Hancock Matt., 'Health Secretary Sets Out Government 'Battle Plan' For Covid-19.' 1 March 2020. https://www.gov.uk/government/news/health-secretary-sets-out-government-battle-plan-for-covid-19. Accessed 14 April 2023.

Hancock, Matt. 'Health and Social Care Secretary's Statement on Coronavirus (COVID-19)' 28 April 2020. https://www.gov.uk/government/speeches/health-and-social-care-secretarys-statement-on-coronavirus-covid-19-28-april-2020. Accessed 14 April 2023.

Hancock, Matt, 'Oral statement on coronavirus and the government's plans for winter.' 17 September 2020 https://www.gov.uk/government/speeches/oral-statement-on-coronavirus-and-the-governments-plans-for-winter. accessed 14 April 2023.

Halifax, Stuart. '"Over by Christmas": British popular opinion and the short war in 1914.' *War Studies* 1:2 (2010), 103–121.

Hansen, Per Krogh. 'Illness and Heroics: On Counter-Narrative And Counter-Metaphor In The Discourse On Cancer.' *Frontiers of Narrative Studies* 4:1 (2018): 213–228.

Hodge, Dan. 'The Left's Hate Mob Can't Stand That Boris Worked Himself Into Intensive Care To Fight (Yes, Fight!) This Virus.' *The Daily Mail*, 12 April 2020. https://www.dailymail.co.uk/debate/article-8211341/The-Lefts-hate-mob-stand-Boris-worked-intensive-care-fight-virus.html. Accessed 14 April 2023.

Hyde, Marina. '"Over by Christmas": Now Where Have We Heard Johnson's New Slogan Before?' *Guardian*, 17 July 2020.https://www.theguardian.com/commentisfree/2020/jul/17/christmas-johnson-slogan-prime-minister-pmqs. Accessed 14 April 2023.

Horton, Richard. 'Offline: COVID-19 as culture war'. *Lancet* 399:10322, (2022) 364.

Johnson, Boris. Prime Minister's statement on coronavirus (COVID-19).' 17 March 2020. https://www.gov.uk/government/speeches/pm-statement-on-coronavirus-17-march-2020

Johnson, Boris. 'Prime Minister's statement on coronavirus (COVID-19).' 10 May 2020. https://www.gov.uk/government/speeches/pm-address-to-the-nation-on-coronavirus-10-may-2020

Johnson, Boris. 'PM speech in Greenwich.' 3 February 2020. https://www.gov.uk/government/speeches/pm-speech-in-greenwich-3-february-2020> Accessed 14 April 2023.

Kahan, Dan. 'Protecting or Polluting the Science Communication Environment?: The Case of Childhood Vaccines.' In *The Oxford Handbook of the Science of Science Communication*, edited by Jamieson, Kathleen Hall., Dan M. Kahan and Dietram A. Scheufele, 422–432. Oxford: Oxford University Press, 2017.

Kohlt, Franziska. "Over by Christmas": The Impact Of War-Metaphors And Other Science-Religion Narratives On Science Communication Environments During The Covid-19 Crisis.' Preprint. SocArXiv. November 2020. https://doi.org/10.31235/osf.io/z5s6a.

Kowol, Kit. 'Britain's Obsession With The Second World War And The Debates That Fuel It.' *The Conversation*, 4 June 2020. https://theconversation.com/britains-obsession-with-the-second-world-war-and-the-debates-that-fuel-it-139497. Accessed 14 April 2023.

Lawson, Nigel. *The View from No.11: Memoirs of a Tory Radical*. London: Bantam Press, 1992.

Maerker, Anna. 'Hagiography and Biography: Narratives of 'Great Men of Science.' In *History, Memory and Public Life: The Past in the Present* edited by Adam Sutcliffe and Simmon Sleight. London: Routledge, 2018.

McGonagle, Emmet. 'Queen's Virus Message On London's Piccadilly Lights Wins Plaudits.' *Campaign*, 9 April 2020. https://www.campaignlive.co.uk/article/queens-virus-message-londons-piccadilly-lights-wins-plaudits/1679849. Accessed 14 April 2023.

Mede, Niels and Mike S Schäfer. 'Science-related Populism: Conceptualizing Populist Demands Toward Science.' *Public Understanding of Science* 29:5 (2020): 473–491.

Middleton, Joe. 'Teachers should be prepared to "sacrifice their lives", says ex-Ofsted head.' *Independent*, 26 February 2021. https://www.independent.co.uk/news/education/covid-schools-reopening-ofsted-teachers-b1807935.html. Accessed 14 April 2023.

Midgley, Mary. *Science as Salvation*. London: Routledge, 2018.

Nie, Jing-Bao., Adam Gilbertson, Malcolm de Roubaix, Ciara Staunton, Anton van Niekerk, Joseph D Tucker and Stuart Rennie, 'Healing Without Waging War: Beyond Military Metaphors in Medicine and HIV Cure Research.' *American Journal for Bioethics* 10 (2016): 3–11. https://doi.org/10.1080/15265161.2016.1214305;

Noakes, Lucy and Juliette Pattinson, '"Keep Calm And Carry On": The Cultural Memory Of The Second World War In Britain.' In *British Cultural Memory and the Second World War*, eds. Lucy Noakes and Juliette Pattinson, 47–66. London: Bloomsbury, 2013.

Okwonga, Musa. 'You cannot sing "Rule Britannia" to a Virus.' *Byline Times*, 19 March 2020. https://bylinetimes.com/2020/03/19/you-cannot-sing-rule-britannia-to-a-virus/. Accessed 14 April 2023.

Panzeri, Francesca., Simona Di Paola, and Filippo Domaneschi, 'Does the COVID-19 War Metaphor Influence Reasoning?' *PLOS One* 24: 3 (2021). https://doi.org/10.1371/journal.pone.0250651.

Pigott, Anna. 'Hocus Pocus? Spirituality And Soil Care In Biodynamic Agriculture.' *EPE: Nature and Space*, 4:4, (2021): 1665–1686.

Pearce, Julia M., G James Rubin, Richard Amlôt, Simon Wessely, and M Brooke Rogers, 'Communicating Public Health Advice After a Chemical Spill: Results From National Surveys in the United Kingdom and Poland.' *Disaster Medicine and Public Health Preparedness* 7:1 (2013), 65–74. https://doi.org/10.1001/dmp.2012.56.

Alec Ryrie, 'Our Sacred Story.' BBC iPlayer, 7 November 2020. https://www.bbc.co.uk/programmes/m000p60n. Accessed 14 April 2023.

Singler, Beth., '"Blessed By The Algorithm": Theistic Conceptions Of Artificial Intelligence In Online Discourse.' *AI & Soc* 35 (2020): 945–955.

Segal, Judy Z., 'Cancer Experience and its Narration: An Accidental Study.' *Literature and Medicine* 30:2 (2012): 292–318.

Segal, Judy Z. *Health and the Rhetoric of Medicine*. Carbondale: Southern Illinois University Press, 2008.

Snape, Michael. *God and the British Soldier: Religion and the British Army in the First and Second World War*. London and New York: Routledge, 2005.

Summer, Michel. 'Willibrord as a Political Actor Between Early Medieval Ireland, Britain and Merovingian Francia (658-739).' (PHD Thesis, Trinity College Dublin, 2021).https://mittelalter.hypotheses.org/26492. Accessed 14 April 2023.

Taylor AJP, *The Origins of the Second World War* (London: Penguin, 1991).

Watson, Janet. 'Total war And Total Anniversary: The Material Culture Of Second World War Commemoration In Britain.' In *Cultural Memory and the Second World War*, eds Lucy Noakes and Juliette Pattinson,175–194. London: Bloomsbury, 2013.

Wessely, Simon and Jo Daniels. 'Why Reassuring The Public May Not Be The Best Way To End Lockdown.' KCL, 9 May 2020. https://www.kcl.ac.uk/news/why-reassuring-the-public-may-not-be-the-best-way-to-end-lockdown. Accessed 14 April 2023.

Wise, Adina. 'The Rhetoric Of War Implies A Heedless Approach That Undermines The Practice Of Medicine.' 17 April 2020. https://blogs.scientificamerican.com/observations/military-metaphors-distort-the-reality-of-covid-19/. Accessed 14 April 2023.

Darren R. Reid

Chapter Seven
"Like i Was in a Movie": Narrative Relativism and Autobiography in the Lockdown Era

Lockdown was a time for storytelling. Prevented from leaving their homes, except for exercise and other essential activities, millions found themselves facing a world increasingly defined by the limits of their accommodation. Responding to the unprecedented, story and storytelling seemed to become all the more important. The sales of books ballooned; digital streaming services became even more ubiquitous; sales of interactive media (particularly videogames) surged; and narratives of national and international unity became common features on daily news broadcasts.[1] In turn, ordinary people became storytellers, as well as consumers of narratives. In person and across social media, they shared and contributed to stories that sought to bring a sense of order to the chaotic reality that accompanied the outbreak. Some looked to grand conspiracy theories.[2] Others looked inward, telling stories about the ways in which lockdown had changed them and their relationship to the wider world.[3]

In the United Kingdom, Prime Minister Boris Johnson un-ironically compared himself to the hapless mayor in Steven Spielberg's *Jaws* (1975).[4] In the Whitehouse,

---

1 Alison Flood, 'UK Book Sales Soared in 2020 Despite Pandemic,' *The Guardian*, 27 April 2020, https://www.theguardian.com/books/2021/apr/27/uk-book-sales-soared-in-2020-despite-pandemic, accessed 8 February 2023; Matt Perez, 'U.S. Video Game Sales Set Record Second Quarter, Spurred by Pandemic,' *Forbes*, 10 August 2020, https://www.forbes.com/sites/mattperez/2020/08/10/video-games-set-record-second-quarter-spurred-by-pandemic-sales/?sh=5aa346ef6f4e, accessed 8 February 2023.; Anon., 'TV Watching and Online Streaming Surge During Lockdown,' *BBC News*, 5 August 2020, https://www.bbc.co.uk/news/entertainment-arts-53637305, accessed 8 February 2023.
2 Philip Ball and Amy Maxmen, 'The Epic Battle against Coronavirus Misinformation and Conspiracy Theories,' *Nature*, 27 May 2020, https://www.nature.com/articles/d41586-020-01452-z, accessed 8 February 2023.
3 Kirsty Grant, 'Covid: Lessons I Learned from Lockdowns in 2020,' *BBC News*, 5 January 2021, https://www.bbc.co.uk/news/newsbeat-54791791, accessed 8 February 2023.
4 Heather Stewart, 'Cummings Brought to Life What Many Already Knew About Johnson's Failures,' *The Guardian*, 26 May 2021, https://www.theguardian.com/politics/2021/may/26/cummings-brought-to-life-what-many-already-knew-about-johnsons-failures, accessed 8 February 2023; Andrew Woodcock, '"Disastrous" Mistakes Caused Tens of Thousands of Unnecessary Deaths from Covid, says Dominic Cummings' *The Independent*, 26 May 2021, https://www.independent.co.uk/

https://doi.org/10.1515/9783110731002-008

then-president Donald J. Trump was telling an increasingly assured-sounding narrative about Chinese laboratories that hinted at biological warfare.[5] And across the wider population, people sought narrative frames which could help them to understand and rationalise the unprecedented. They contacted loved ones and peers, speculating and hunting for appropriate narratives. They participated in the generation of communal tales: 'Rumours', as one *#RecordCovid19* correspondent put it, 'were starting to circulate'.[6] Millions of parents had to explain to their children why the fundamental paradigm of their lives had had to undergo such a sudden and radical transformation. Family members and friends sought comfort in each other, reminiscing about better, freer times.[7] Romantic partners shared photographs and anecdotes online, celebrating the companionship which (they hoped) would sustain them throughout the crisis.[8] Later, stories were told about rising divorce rates; or the overlooked victims of domestic abuse whose lives were made immeasurably worse by the sudden imposition of a lockdown that left them trapped with an abusive spouse, partner, parent, or carer.[9]

In the lockdown-era, the boundary between the tellers and consumers of stories became blurred, a reality that must profoundly impact how we remember, memorialise, and come to terms with these events.[10] To understand lockdown,

---

news/uk/politics/dominic-cummings-covid-boris-johnson-b1854048.html, accessed 8 February 2023.

5 Dan Mangan, 'Trump Blames China for Coronavirus Pandemic: "The World is Paying a Very Big Price for What They Did', *CNBC*, 19 March 2020, https://www.cnbc.com/2020/03/19/coronavi rus-outbreak-trump-blames-china-for-virus-again.html, accessed 8 February 2023.; Anon., 'Coronavirus: Trump Stands by China Lab Origin Theory for Virus' *BBC News*, 1 May 2020, https:// www.bbc.co.uk/news/world-us-canada-52496098, accessed 8 February 2023.

6 [*#RecordCovid19*–39] Lincolnshire, Accountant, Male, 23. http://kristopherlovell.com/2020/04/28/ record-covid19-38-lincolnshire-accountant-male-23/, accessed 8 February 2023.

7 [*#RecordCovid19*–53] W. Wales, Freelance Teacher, Trainer Project Manager, Female, 61, http:// kristopherlovell.com/2020/05/11/recordcovid19-53-w-wales-freelance-teacher-trainer-project-man ager-female-61/, accessed 14 April 2023.

8 Kori L. Krueger and Amanda L. Forest, 'Communicating Commitment: A Relationship–Protection Account of Dyadic Displays on Social Media,' *Personality and Social Psychology Bulletin*, 46 (2020): 1059-1073.

9 Maya Oppenheim, 'Divorce Enquiries to Legal Firms Soar by 95% in Pandemic with Women Driving Surge in Interest,' *Independent*, 8 May 2021, https://www.independent.co.uk/news/uk/ home-news/divorce-inquiries-rise-pandemic-women–b1843359.html, accessed 8 February 2023. Gene Feder, Ana Flavia Lucas d'Oliveira, Poonam Risha and Medina Johnson, 'Domestic Violence During the Pandemic.' *BMJ* 372 (2021): n722.

10 There is a broad literature that engages with issues relating to cultural memory and the role of community narrative creation. Though far from an exhaustive list, the following pieces will provide insight into the study of this phenomenon from a number of different cultural perspectives: Jan Assmann, 'Collective Memory and Cultural Identity,' *New German Critique* 65 (1995):

one must prioritise (if not necessarily centre) storytelling within their interpretive framework. To not do so would be to miss a critical aspect of the lived experience of so many: the narratives they consumed to help them to escape or understand their plight; and the stories they told which allowed them to take some degree of control over their lives.[11] The stories shared by individuals were frequently autobiographical in nature, even when many of them sought to retell existing narratives, or were centred upon third parties. When Boris Johnson referenced *Jaws*, he did so in an attempt explain himself, his motivations, and his plans.[12] He was looking to a third-party narrative, to be sure, but was placing himself into a context of its story – a process this piece defines as narrative relativism. Autobiography, be it written or oral, was frequently implied by the types of stories that were told throughout lockdown, and the self was frequently centred.[13]

125–133; Alon Confino, 'Collective Memory and Cultural History: Problems of Method,' *The American Historical Review* 102 (1997): 1386–1403; Susannah Radstone and Bill Schwarz, *Memory: Histories, Theories Debates* (New York: Fordham University Press, 2010); Wulf Kansteiner, 'Finding Meaning in Memory: A Methodological Critique of Collective Memory Studies,' *History and Theory* 41 (2002): 179–197.

11 Patrick Ryan, 'The Storyteller in Context: Storyteller Identity and Storytelling Experience,' *Storytelling, Self, Society* 4, (2008): 64-87.

12 Johnson's use of the *Jaws* reference inspired further narratives in the British press as different news organizations sought to rationalize, contextualize, or ignore the Prime Minister's apparently happy self-comparison with one of the most obviously wrongheaded politicians in mainstream fiction. *The Guardian* newspaper wrote sarcastically about what it portended for the future; *The Independent* was incredulous; The *Daily Express* was largely neutral; Whilst *BBC News* was conspicuously quiet, largely ignoring the issue. See Stuart Heritage, 'Boris Johnson's Hero is the Mayor Who Kept the Beaches Open in Jaws. That's Fine By Me,' *The Guardian*, 13 March 2020, https://www.theguardian.com/film/2020/mar/13/boris-johnson-coronavirus-hero-mayor-larry-vaughn-jaws, accessed 8 February 2023; Tim Wyatt, 'Boris Johnson Has History of Comparing Himself to Jaws' Reckless Mayor Who Kept Beaches Open,' *The Independent*, 27 April 2021, https://www.independent.co.uk/news/uk/politics/boris-johnson-jaws-mayor-beach-b1838049.html, accessed 14 April 2023; Martina Bet, 'Coronavirus Action Plan: How Boris Johnson Said "He is Inspired by Mayor from Jaws,"' *The Independent*, 13 March 2020, https://www.express.co.uk/news/uk/1254769/coronavirus-uk-news-cases-deaths-schools-boris-johnson-strategy-jaws-major-spt, accessed 8 February 2023. The only time the BBC appeared to engage with this issue (contemporaneously) was on 26 May 2021, when Dominic Cummings gave evidence against the government's handling of the initial coronavirus crisis. In that article, the mention appears briefly in a bullet-point summary of Cummings's allegations. The article offers no analysis of the accusation, nor any further insight. See 'Covid: Boris Johnson's "Bodies Pile High" Comments Prompt Criticism,' *BBC News*, 26 April 2021, https://www.bbc.co.uk/news/uk-politics-56890714, accessed 8 February 2023.

13 For discussions about some of the problematizing issues which affect autobiography see Anthony Palmer and T.S. Champlin, 'Self–Deception: A Problem about Autobiography,' *Proceedings of the Aristotelian Society, Supplementary Volumes* 53 (1979): 61–94; Michael Sprinker, 'Fictions of the Self: The End of Autobiography,' in *Autobiography: Essays Theoretical and Critical*, ed. James

#RecordCovid19 is one of several source-bases which captures the autobiographical trend and narrative relativism present in so much lockdown storytelling, as well as the importance of interpretative frameworks created by the repurposing of existing narratives. As such, it must necessarily bring to mind issues and debates connected with the use of oral history, another autobiographical form of primary evidence which tends to capture subjective, self-curated reminisces.[14] The accounts in *#RecordCovid19* are not oral histories in the traditional sense. They were primarily written documents, but in a digital age which allows for near-instantaneous written communication, and the swift collection of self-curated personal narratives, they are functionally very similar. As such they are prone to many of the same concerns and benefits which affect other forms of oral history.[15] That is to say, they are not necessarily sources one should consult in order to find facts, but they are the types of sources which provide scholars and commentators with an insight into how facts were interpreted, internalised, and understood by contemporaries.[16] So many of the ad hoc autobiographies created by lockdown were ephemeral in nature, told in one-off conversations as people reflected upon the changes lockdown had imposed upon their lives. *#RecordCovid19* and its peers provided mechanisms through which some portion of these self-curated reflections can be preserved and studied.[17]

For many, storytelling and narrative construction was an essential part of the lockdown experience. Stories provided interpretative frameworks to understand the exceptional; they provided a device for communities to build a common dialogue; and they provided opportunities for autobiographical reflection.[18] *#RecordCovid19* and other such source-bases are, like all primary sources, far from problem-free, but they are also opportunity-rich. The subjective and autobiographical nature of these sources is not necessarily a problem for scholars, so long as the sources are

---

Olney (Princeton: Princeton University Press, 1980), 321–342; Charles Berryman, 'Critical Mirrors: Theories of Autobiography,' *Mosaic: An Interdisciplinary Critical Journal* 32 (1999): 71-84.

14 For discussions on the use of comparable sources, particularly the role played by autobiography in oral history, see Alistair Thomson, 'Oral History and Community History in Britain: Personal and Critical Reflections on Twenty–Five Years of Continuity and Change,' *Oral History* 36 (2008): 95–104; Shelley Trower, 'Auto/Biographical Oral Histories, from "Oral Memories" to "The Life of Nate Shaw,"' *Oral History* 45 (2017): 43–45; Joanna Bornat, 'Oral History and Remembering,' in *Research Methods for Memory Studies*, eds. Emily Keightley and Michael Pickering (Edinburgh: Edinburgh University Press, 2013), 29–42.

15 Paul Thomson, *The Voice of the Past: Oral History* (Oxford: Oxford University Press, 1988), 28.

16 Lynn Abrams, *Oral History Theory* (London and New York: Routledge, 2016), 58-78.

17 For examples of other Covid-19 oral history projects, see 'Covid-19 Oral History Project': https://covid-19archive.org; 'Covid-19 & Me', https://libguides.princeton.edu/c.php?g=937179&p=7407469; and 'The Irish COVID–19 Oral History Project', https://covid19oralhistory.ie.

18 Sherif Hetata, 'The Self and Autobiography,' *PMLA* 118 (2003): 123-125.

used with care and the storytelling mechanisms which informed them are under-stood and integrated into a careful analysis of these accounts.

Narrative Relativism

There was an inherent sense of mystery to the virus which defied most peoples' prior lived experience. 'When I first heard about it on Youtube', one respondent wrote, 'I heard it kills . . . in twenty-four hours.'[19] Others 'heard about it on the news', internalising vague stories about a 'deadly virus in China' which, at this stage in the pandemic, lacked any real detail.[20] Some respondents to #RecordCovid19 reported being 'haunted by the virus' or contemplating a future in which some form of lock down, the 'new normal', was here to stay: 'will this ever end?'[21] This sense of uncertainty was reflected in rapid changes to real-world behaviours. As news of the virus spread, alongside rumours of lockdowns, supermarket shelves were emptied of food and other essential items. In the West, where such items are rarely, if ever, in short supply, the sight was shocking.[22] Social media times were quickly populated by negative stories about panic-buyers: 'What barbarity! What ignorance! Can they even be called human . . . these [words] pretty much sum up what some of my social media "friends" posted in reaction to the news.'[23] In the early phase of the pandemic, where accurate information was scarce and 'panic' common, the sudden disappearance of toilet paper and pasta from store shelves prompted many to look beyond real world experiences.[24] As

---

19 [*#RecordCovid19*–38] Turkey, Student, Female, 18, http://kristopherlovell.com/2020/04/28/re cord-covid19-37-turkey-student-female-18/, accessed 14 April 2023, accessed 14 April 2023.
20 [*#RecordCovid19*–105] Birmingham, Student, Male, 21, http://kristopherlovell.com/2020/12/23/re cordcovid19-105-birmingham-united-kingdom-male-21–student/, accessed 14 April 2023.
21 [*#RecordCovid19*–52] London, Civil Servant, 25-30, http://kristopherlovell.com/2020/05/11/re cordcovid19-52-london-civil-servant-25-30/, accessed 14 April 2023; [*#RecordCovid19*–60] Sweden, Sick Leave, Male, 27, http://kristopherlovell.com/2020/05/26/recordcovid19-60-sweden-sick-leave-male-27-yo/, accessed 14 April 2023.
22 [*#RecordCovid19*–105] Birmingham, Student, Male, 21, http://kristopherlovell.com/2020/12/23/re cordcovid19-105-birmingham-united-kingdom-male-21-student/, accessed 14 April 2023.
23 [*#RecordCovid19*–31] Istanbul, Turkey, Undergraduate Student, Female, 41, http://kristopherlo vell.com/2020/04/27/record-covid19-31-istanbul-turkey-undergraduate-student-female–41/, accessed 14 April 2023.
24 [*#RecordCovid19*–95] Cambridge (UK), University Employee, Male, 25-34, http://kristopherlo vell.com/2020/10/07/recordcovid19-95-cambridge-uk-university-employee-male-25-34/, accessed 14 April 2023; [*#RecordCovid19*–105] Birmingham, Student, Male, 21, http://kristopherlovell.com/ 2020/12/23/recordcovid19-105-birmingham-united-kingdom-male-21-student/, accessed 14 April

one respondent put it, 'I felt like I was in a movie. A drama movie [where] people die.'[25]

The perceived unreality of lockdown fuelled such narrative relativism. One respondent, reflecting on the fear that accompanied the initial spread of the disease, described life as feeling 'like a horror movie'.[26] Another noted that '[t]he surreal feeling was overwhelming' and that 'it was like [being] in a sci-fi film'.[27] Yet another, watching the early spread of the virus in northern Italy (February-March 2020), felt as if they were watching the unfolding of 'some kind of zombie-plot'.[28] One even looked to Disney/Pixar for an appropriate narrative device: 'I feel like I'm in the incinerator from Toy Story 3'.[29] The parallels being drawn with works of fiction should not be surprising. Disaster narratives have been a popular genre for decades with popular entries in that canon appearing frequently in the lead-up to the outbreak. To name just a few: *Outbreak* (1995), *Resident Evil* (1996–present), *28 Days Later* (2002), *The Day After Tomorrow* (2004), *Dawn of the Dead* (2004), *Cloverfield* (2008), *2012* (2009), *Zombieland* (2009), *The Walking Dead* (2010–2022), *The Last of Us* (2013), *World War Z* (2013), *Godzilla* (2014), *Extinction* (2018), *Bird Box* (2018), and *The Dead Don't Die* (2019). Whilst most of these films were fantastical and did not reflect the precise circumstances faced by respondents during the pandemic, many of them contained moments, scenes, or settings that became particularly relatable after the outbreak of the pandemic: the collapse of supply chains, widespread panic, social isolation, and the need to significantly modify one's behaviour to improve their odds of survival. These fictive reference points were important, but they did not necessarily promote hopelessness, despite their rather grim settings. Many of them are, after all, ultimately stories of survival. As one respondent put it, 'it felt like we were all part of an apocalyptic movie but [it was] weirdly comforting that everyone all

2023; [#RecordCovid19–31] Istanbul, Turkey, Undergraduate Student, Female, 41, http://kristo pherlovell.com/2020/04/27/record-covid19-31-istanbul-turkey-undergraduate-student-female-41/, accessed 14 April 2023.

25 *[#RecordCovid19–36]* Turkey, Student, Female, 20, http://kristopherlovell.com/2020/04/28/re cord-covid19-36-turkey-student-female-20/, accessed 14 April 2023.

26 [#RecordCovid19–38] Turkey, Student, Female, 18, http://kristopherlovell.com/2020/04/28/re cord-covid19-37-turkey-student-female-18/, accessed 14 April 2023.

27 [#RecordCovid19–39] Lincolnshire, accountant, male, 23, http://kristopherlovell.com/2020/04/ 28/record-covid19-38-lincolnshire-accountant-male-23/, accessed 14 April 2023.

28 [#RecordCovid19–77] England, Student, 20, http://kristopherlovell.com/2020/09/13/recordco vid19-77-20-student-england/, accessed 14 April 2023.

29 [#RecordCovid19–51] Suffolk, England, Postgraduate Student, Female, 22, http://kristopherlovell. com/2020/05/11/recordcovid19-51-suffolk-england-postgrad-student-female-22/, accessed 14 April 2023.

over the world [was] going through the same thing at the same time[,] creating a universal experience'.[30]

Respondents to *#RecordCovid19* evidenced the importance external narrative devices. Those devices did not, however, become an obsession and the narrative relativism occasioned by lockdown remained focused on memories of pre-pandemic content. Whilst Steven Soderbergh's *Contagion* (2011), a relatively minor hit upon its initial release, found renewed success after the start of lockdown, the most successful entertainment products of the lockdown-era offered an escape rather than an echo chamber.[31] *Tiger King* (2020), a rather ridiculous documentary series about one man's love, and exploitation, of tigers was the breakout hit of early-lockdown, whilst family-fare, such as *The Croods 2: A New Age* (2020), performed admirably well throughout the second half of the year.[32] In the second wave of lockdowns, consumer entertainment remained reliably escapist in nature. Disney's staple of Marvel-based content –*WandaVision* (2021), *The Falcon and the Winter Soldier* (2021), and *Loki* (2021)– proved to be a significant hit with viewers.[33] In some cases, entertainment offered unintentional parallels to the pandemic that occasioned little, if any, contemporary comment. Disney's *The Mandalorian* (2019-present), a show set in the *Star Wars* universe, told the story of a man coming to terms with having to remove a mask that had hitherto defined his life, a narrative device that could have, but did not seem to, impact contentious debates about mask-wearing and post-lockdown adjustments. For the most part, audiences of *The Mandalorian* were so enamoured with its characters and setting than they seemed uninterested in the

---

30 [*#RecordCovid19*–91] Coventry, Student, Female, 19, http://kristopherlovell.com/2020/10/05/recordcovid19-91-coventry-student-female-19/, accessed 14 April 2023.

31 Brandon Katz, 'The 10 Most Watched Movies on Netflix During Lockdown,' *The Observer*, 21 April 2020, https://observer.com/2020/04/netflix-ratings-most-watched-movies-what-to-stream-covid-19, accessed 8 February 2023; David Fear, 'How "Contagion" Suddenly Became the Most Urgent Movie of 2020,' *Rolling Stone*, 13 March 2020, https://www.rollingstone.com/movies/movie-features/contagion-most-urgent-movie-of-2020-964532, accessed 8 February 2023; Rebecca Nicholson, 'Insane, Intoxicating Tiger King is Perfect Lockdown TV,' *The Guardian*, 4 April 2020, https://www.theguardian.com/commentisfree/2020/apr/04/insane-intoxicating-tale-of-big-cats-is-perfect-lockdown-tv-tiger-watch-james-mcavoy-greta-gerwig, accessed 8 February 2023; Christopher Palm and Lucas Shaw, '"Tiger King" Documentary a Netflix Hit in Coronavirus Lockdown,' *Bloomberg*, 8 April 2020, https://www.bloomberg.com/news/articles/2020-04-08/netflix-s-quirky-tiger-king-becomes-breakout-pandemic-hit, accessed 8 February 2023.

32 Scott Mendelson, 'Box Office: "Soul" Nabs $6M in China as "Croods 2" Nears $100M Global,' *Forbes*, 27 December 2020: https://www.forbes.com/sites/scottmendelson/2021/12/27/box-office-soul-nabs-6m-in-china-as-croods-2-nears-100m-global/?sh=7e95904c327a, accessed 8 February 2023.

33 Paul Tassi, '"Loki" Hits #1 Globally Faster than "Falcon" or "WandaVision" on Disney Plus,' *Forbes*, 19 June 2021, https://www.forbes.com/sites/paultassi/2021/06/19/loki-hits-1-globally-faster-than-falcon-or-wandavision-on-disney-plus/?sh=4a6755333c36, accessed 8 February 2023.

ways that its main character's struggle seemed to parallel real world discourses.[34] There was little appetite for audiences to project the current pandemic onto a galaxy far, far away.

If lockdown-era entertainment offered an escape, pre-lockdown narratives offered precedent. Beyond zombie and disaster movies, *#RecordCovid19* shows how the popular memory of historic episodes could provide a framework of understanding. In Britain, a 'blitz spirit' narrative quickly emerged that heralded back to popular images of the country during the Second World War.[35] As one respondent put it, 'I don't think I ever understood the rather deep relationship between a Prime Minister and the state of public attitude during war, or [other] times of great strain'.[36] This respondent was almost certainly referencing the Churchillian trope so popular in modern British culture.[37] Across the British media a 'blitz spirit' narrative had emerged during the first lockdown that harkened back to a grossly over-simplified narrative of wartime unity. In reality, the Second World War was a period in which internal conflict and disagreement was common in Great Britain; realities which subsequent generations have largely cleansed from popular memory. Whilst broad unity and a self-sacrificing spirit was present at times, that was not always the case.[38] Such nuance had little place in the 'blitz spirit' narrative, however. The same respondent as above would marvel at the ways in which the apparent spirit of the

---

34 For examples that are broadly representative of *The Mandalorian*'s critical reception, see Laura Prudom, 'The Mandalorian: Season 2 Review,' *IGN*, 23 December 2020, https://www.ign.com/articles/the-mandalorian-season-2-review, accessed 8 February 2023; Tyler Hersko, '"The Mandalorian" Review: Season 2 Ends with a Noisy, Mindless Slaughter,' *IndieWire*, 18 December 2020, https://www.indiewire.com/2020/12/the-mandalorian-review-season-2-finale-1234605624, accessed 8 February 2023; Rebecca Harrison, 'The Mandalorian Season 2 Seeks Hope in a Bruised and Battered Galaxy,' *BFI*, 21 December 2020, https://www.bfi.org.uk/sight-and-sound/reviews/mandalorian-season-2-star-wars-spin-off-disney-grogu-din-djarin, accessed 8 February 2023.
35 Anon., 'Spirit of the Blitz,' *The Economist*, 21 March 2020, https://www.economist.com/britain/2020/03/21/spirit-of-the-blitz, accessed 14 April 2023; Richard Overy, 'Why the Cruel Myth of the "Blitz Spirit" is No Model for How to Fight Coronavirus,' *The Guardian*, 19 March 2020, https://www.theguardian.com/commentisfree/2020/mar/19/myth-blitz-spirit-model-coronavirus, accessed 8 February 2023.; Katherine Dunn, 'To Tackle Coronavirus, Brits are Appealing to an Age-Old Rallying Cry: "Blitz Spirit,"' *Fortune*, 6 March 2020, https://fortune.com/2020/03/06/coronavirus-brexit-blitz-spirit, accessed 8 February 2023.
36 [#RecordCovid19–43] Student, Female, 20, http://kristopherlovell.com/2020/05/01/record-covid19-43-student-female–20/, accessed 8 February 2023.
37 Alma Pierre Bonnet, 'The "Churchill Factor" and Its Influence On The Brexit Debate: Defining The Churchill Myth,' *Observatoire de la Société Britannique 25 (2020), 65–86*.
38 Darren Kelsey, 'The Myth of the "Blitz Spirit" in British Newspaper Responses to the July 7th Bombings,' *Social Semiotics* 23 (2013): 83–99; Siân Nicholas, 'History, Revisionism, and Television Drama: Foyle's War and the "Myth of 1940,"' *Media History* 13 (2007): 203–219.

moment had reshaped their relationship with politics: 'I honestly never thought I'd be waiting each day to see a figure like Boris Johnson or Dominic Raab speak at a podium, and yet here I am'.[39]

As discussed by Kristopher Lovell in Chapter One, respondents from a variety of countries dwelled upon the historic nature of the moment; that they were participants in the type of grand narratives about which they had previously only read but never experienced, something their 'children and grand-children would read about in their history textbooks'.[40] Despite the perceived historical significance of the pandemic, however, the past was typically invoked in an abstract way by respondents, with few offering specific historic parallels or comparisons. In all of *#RecordCovid19*, there were, only two references to the Spanish Flu, despite that outbreak being a prominent part of the media discourse during the early stage of the pandemic.[41] The coronavirus was referred to on several occasions as a 'plague' (or even, 'the plague'), but even that label tended to lack significant historicism with one respondent using the word to relate the virus with zombies, not past outbreaks of disease.[42] Despite this relative lack of specificity, history nonetheless provided a framework that allowed many to understand the scale of what was happening around them – and to order and communicate their thoughts on those events.

---

39 [*#RecordCovid19*–43] Student, Female, 20, http://kristopherlovell.com/2020/05/01/record-covid19-43-student-female-20/, accessed 14 April 2023.

40 [*#RecordCovid19*–39] Lincolnshire, Accountant, Male, 23, http://kristopherlovell.com/2020/04/28/record-covid19-38-lincolnshire-accountant-male-23/, accessed 14 April 2023.

41 [*#RecordCovid19*–26] Newport South Wales, MA Student, http://kristopherlovell.com/2020/04/25/record-covid19-26-newport-south-wales-ma-student-female-22/, accessed 14 April 2023; [*#RecordCovid19*–7] UK, Writer, Male, 18+. http://kristopherlovell.com/2020/04/14/record-covid-19-7-uk-writer-male-18/, accessed 14 April 2023.

42 For examples of uses of the word 'plague' (or 'the plague') see [*#RecordCovid19*–84] London, Office Worker, Female, 40-Something, http://kristopherlovell.com/2020/10/05/recordcovid19-84-london-office-worker-female-40-something/, accessed 14 April 2023; [*#RecordCovid19*–94] Northeast Florida, Retired Psychologist, Female, 75, http://kristopherlovell.com/2020/10/07/recordcovid19-94-northeast-florida-75-year-old-female-retired-psychologist/, accessed 14 April 2023; [*#RecordCovid19*–75] UK, Unemployed, Female, 28, http://kristopherlovell.com/2020/07/19/recordcovid19-74-uk-unemployed-the-current-national-occupation-female-28/, accessed 14 April 2023; [*#RecordCovid19*–77] England, Student, 20, http://kristopherlovell.com/2020/09/13/recordcovid19-77-20-student-england/. For examples of 'plague' being linked to medieval disease outbreaks see [*#RecordCovid19*–24] Sweden, Sick Leave, Male, 27, http://kristopherlovell.com/2020/04/24/record-covid19-24-sweden-sick-leave-27m/, accessed 14 April 2023; [*#RecordCovid19*–26] Newport South Wales, MA student, Female: 25 April 2020, http://kristopherlovell.com/2020/04/25/record-covid19-26-newport-south-wales-ma-student-female-22/, accessed 14 April 2023.

Narrative frameworks changed over time, however. In the UK, the 'blitz spirit' narrative unravelled with the end of the first lockdown (see Christopher Smith's chapter for more). Writing in April 2020, a British shop assistant reflected on the positive change that lockdown had had upon his customers. '[O]n the whole,' he wrote, 'customers have adopted these to changes fantastically. Very few of them have complained, although many have acted forgetfully over the social distancing procedures . . . Personally, it has been heart-warming and encouraging that a significant number of people are "thanking us for staying open" or even just telling us to "stay safe".'[43] Within a few weeks of writing this, however, #RecordCovid19 shows how, even in the context of the 'blitz spirit' narrative, differing ideas about acceptable lockdown behaviour were beginning to manifest themselves. 'This country makes me sick', wrote one correspondent. They went on to explain: 'Yesterday was VE Day and the news coverage of people just abandoning everything and having street parties is astounding. Don't get me wrong, I'm not a fan of nationalist, jingoistic BS at the best of times, but there's a depressing irony about people getting together to celebrate the sacrifices of others whilst refusing to do the same themselves. I can't help but wonder how many people will suffer as a result of this, or how many would have been saved if it was raining yesterday.'[44] As government messaging changed, becoming more divisive, further strain was placed upon the united 'blitz spirit' narrative. 'I'm glad I live in Wales,' wrote one, 'Boris Johnson has just spoken of lifting some of the restrictions in England, and now the slogan is "stay alert, control the virus, save lives". Which is yet another example of the rock solid, completely unmistakable guidance with no room whatsoever for varied and conflicting interpretations'. Lest the tone of their writing be mistaken, they sought to clarify their view on government policy: 'it is flimsier than a filo pastry'.[45]

Changes in government messaging shattered illusions of togetherness and, with it, the 'blitz spirit' narrative began to crumble: 'I feel like I'm in [an] incinerator, trying desperately to run from a massive fiery hole, and someone's at the controls, and everyone's screaming for them to do something and they're just singing Vera Bloody Lynn as though if we were all a little more gung-ho and Blitz Spirited about this then we'd all be muddling along nicely. I hate that our country is nearly the

---

43 [*#RecordCovid19*–29] Bridgnorth, Shop Assistant, Male, 24, http://kristopherlovell.com/2020/04/25/record-covid19-29-bridgnorth-shop-assistant-male-24/, accessed 14 April 2023.
44 [*#RecordCovid19*–49] Wales, Engineer, Female, 30, http://kristopherlovell.com/2020/05/09/record-covid19-49-wales-engineer-female-30/, accessed 14 April 2023.
45 [*#RecordCovid19*–5] Wales, Writer, Female, 28, http://kristopherlovell.com/2020/05/10/recordcovid19-50-wales-writer-female-28/, accessed 14 April 2023.

laughing stock of the world.'[46] *#RecordCovid19* shows a marked increase in its respondents' agitation around May 10th, the date that Boris Johnson announced the easing of lockdown restrictions in the UK. As one respondent put it: 'I can't sleep. Earlier today (although it's actually the day after at time of writing) Prime Minister Boris 'Take It On The Chin' Johnson spoke in a pre[-]recorded speech about steps moving forward. It has become clear, or at least it feels clear to me that we are nowhere near ready . . . tonight the government have even taken sleep from me.'[47] With government policy no longer enjoying broad support, criticism of politicians in *#RecordCovid19* increased. 'I hate the fact that any semblance of democracy seems to have disappeared', wrote one, the day after Johnson's speech.[48] The perceived 'hypocrisy displayed by the UK government' created a furious response among those respondents who believed the government was acting prematurely and without due haste or care.[49] 'This is the first time I have cried with rage', wrote a respondent, 'I want to throw things at the wall and watch them break. If I could leave the house, I'd get on the first train I could and beat down the doors of Downing Street with my fists. I'd break my own bones against the walls of government if I had to. But I can't do that.'[50] By the end of the year, and with the approach of another lockdown, the 'blitz spirit' narrative had evaporated completely: 'The mood of the country definitely feels to have changed. During the first lockdown there was a pulling together, a sense of we're all in this together that I feel is lacking now . . . we're not all in this together.'[51]

The ultimate failure of the narrative of the 'blitz spirit' was important. Facing the unprecedented, people looked to stories, but their relationship with politically loaded narratives changed as government policy and circumstance began to shift. It is perhaps telling that *#RecordCovid19* captures the disintegration of perceived national unity and the 'blitz spirit', whilst, if anything, that same source-base seems

---

46 [*#RecordCovid19*–51] Suffolk, England, Postgraduate Student, Female, 22, http://kristopherlovell. com/2020/05/11/recordcovid19-51-suffolk-england-postgrad-student-female–22/, accessed 14 April 2023.

47 [*#RecordCovid19*–52] London, Civil Servant, 25–30, http://kristopherlovell.com/2020/05/11/re cordcovid19-52-london-civil-servant-25-30/, accessed 14 April 2023.

48 [*#RecordCovid19*–53] West Wales, Freelance Teacher, Trainer, Project Manager, Female, 61, http://kristopherlovell.com/2020/05/11/recordcovid19-53-w-wales-freelance-teacher-trainer-project-manager-female-61/, accessed 14 April 2023.

49 [*#RecordCovid19*–56] Wales, Engineer, Female, 30, http://kristopherlovell.com/2020/05/26/re cordcovid19-56-wales-engineer-female-30/, accessed 14 April 2023.

50 [*#RecordCovid19*-57] Wales, Writer, Female, 28, http://kristopherlovell.com/2020/05/26/recordco vid19-57-wales-writer-female-28/, accessed 14 April 2023.

51 [*#RecordCovid19*–100] Brierfield, East Lancashire, Recently Unemployed, Male, 39, http://kristo pherlovell.com/2020/11/01/recordcovid19-100-brierfield-east-lancashire-recently-unemployed-male-39/, accessed 14 April 2023.

to suggest that, as the crisis began to ease and respondents were increasingly minded to look back on it as a historic episode, that apocalyptic works of fiction and zombie movies remained fond points of reference.[52] To be sure, more research will be needed in the years and decades to come in order to confirm this phenomena, but the catastrophic collapse of a narrative of national unity in the face of fantastic images of the walking dead, is a remarkable occurrence worthy of further reflection. Perhaps of more immediate concern, however, is the role played by all forms narratives during the pandemic era – and the participatory role taken by ordinary people who became the (re)tellers of such tales.

The Autobiographical Impulse

#RecordCovid19 captured important insights and anecdotes about life during the pandemic – fear, anger, disappointment, boredom, and much more besides. But it also captured something else: an autobiographical storytelling process that was as important and interesting as anything else in the record. Faced with an unprecedented crisis, people looked to narratives (fictive, historical, and otherwise) for frames of reference – and they created their own. From Joseph Campbell to Alex Rosenberg, the importance of the narrative to the human condition has been an important research theme in many fields.[53] In history, this has not always been the case. A.J.P. Taylor's much requoted dismissal of oral history ('old men drooling about their youth') misses a rather important point – that the process of memorialisation and storytelling is fundamental; and understanding how and why narratives are constructed can provide important insights into the lived experiences of one's subjects.[54] To put it simply, the fact that 'old men drool' over their youths is an important observation and understanding why that occurs, and what it means for the creation of shared narratives and myths, is no small matter. Remembering and for-

52 [*#RecordCovid19*–77] England, Student, 20, http://kristopherlovell.com/2020/09/13/recordcovid19-77-20-student-england/, accessed 14 April 2023; [*#RecordCovid19*–91] Coventry, Student, Female, 19, http://kristopherlovell.com/2020/10/05/recordcovid19-91-coventry-student-female–19/, accessed 14 April 2023.
53 Joseph Campbell, *The Hero with a Thousand Faces*, 3rd edition (New York: Pantheon Books, 1949; reprint, Novato: New World Library, 2008), 1–40; Alex Rosenberg *How History Gets Things Wrong: The Neuroscience of Our Addiction to Stories* (Cambridge: MIT Press, 2018), 1–14.
54 Donald A. Ritchie, *Doing Oral History* (Oxford: Oxford University Press, 2015), xiv.

getting are key parts of the historic process and the types of sources that evidence this are important for a number of reasons.[55]

#RecordCovid19 does not contain oral histories – but it does contain ad hoc autobiographies which function in a similar way. The respondents to *#RecordCovid19* were a self-selecting group, formed, at least in part, by their awareness of the project and of a desire to contribute to the historic record. These accounts have been prepared with an audience in mind, and whilst they certainly provide honest and intellectually interesting insights, they are necessarily curated and exclusive. For all the detail they give, much is surely omitted. In many instances, respondents engaged in direct autobiography construction. 'For the record', one respondent wrote, 'I still feel guilty because I am liking (most) of my lockdown / isolationist life. I have just enough work to get by, I have a fantastic house and garden, I have a lot of walks by turning left or right out of my back door'.[56] Others provided insight into their family lives, though these tended to be impressionistic and rather broad in nature: '[t]he hardest part is dealing with the mental health of my family. Some o[f] my family members are almost in a constant panic over covid, fearing death around every corner. Complaining that we should fully isolate ourselves and stop working, only to turn around and have a panic attack over the reduced income.'[57] Such accounts do an admirable job of describing how the family, as a broad unit, was responding to the crisis, without offering specific examples about individual family members and their lived experiences. The details in such accounts is welcome, whilst the excluded information –who felt this way; how their feelings had changed over time; what were the motivating factors behind particular attitudes or actions? – is frequently absent. This should not reflect negatively on any of the respondents. The desire to maintain the privacy of one's family and peers is a common and understandable phenomenon, but it is a reality that nonetheless needs to be acknowledged. As a result of this, *#RecordCovid19* is less a source-base that illustrates how the family and friends of a respondent behaved and thought, and more one which illustrates how the respondents themselves felt about the perceived

---

55 W. Fitzhugh Brundage, 'Commemoration and Conflict: Forgetting and Remembering the Civil War,' *The Georgia Historical Quarterly* 82 (1998): 559–574; Evan Faulkenbury, '"A Problem of Visibility": Remembering and Forgetting the Civil War in Cortland, New York,' *The Public Historian* 41 (2019): 83–99.

56 [*#RecordCovid19*–98] Wales, Freelance Teacher, Trainer, Project Manager, Female, now 62, http://kristopherlovell.com/2020/10/20/recordcovid19-98-west-wales-freelance-teacher-trainer-project-manager-female-now-62/, accessed 14 April 2023.

57 [*#RecordCovid19*–101] Sweden, Office Worker, Male 28, http://kristopherlovell.com/2020/11/02/recordcovid19-101-sweden-office-worker-male-28/, accessed 14 April 2023.

actions and attitudes of those around them. Typically, respondents placed themselves at the centre of their accounts.

At its most explicit, the autobiographical impulse was clear and deliberate. 'I'm a proper introvert', one respondent wrote, '[a]s a rule I keep well away from noisy, sociable folk as I find their kind of "fun", especially organised "fun", quite unbearable. I've always avoided joining-in. Seriously, if I get invited to a gathering, even drinks after work, part of me dies inside. And as for a wedding invitation? Well my heart falls into my boots . . . Will there be dancing? Oh god, no please . . . [s]o, lockdown then? Absolutely fine. I have my books.[58] Other respondents would likewise provide comparable insights their self-image (alongside details of everyday activities): 'Unfortunately I've sunk into the banana bread craze and my small home has no garden, with no access to the outdoors and only baked goods to keep me comfort I'll be lucky to come out of this without rickets. Humour though, has always kept me company.'[59] Even when respondents addressed external events, their entries were frequently more revealing about themselves than anything else. 'Rather than tell my specific COVID-19 story', one respondent wrote, 'I want to record what I was thinking'. The resultant account is a broad summary of events leading up to the first lockdown, reframed, as they themselves acknowledge, by information they gained later – 'what I now know'. Whilst not an account of their 'story', the resulting entry nonetheless provides an insight into that respondent. It seems telling that they identify as a writer, and that they chose to contribute to the record not by telling their own tale, but that of others.[60]

The treatment of the self within *#RecordCovid19* is an important indicator of how individuals dealt with the changing context created by a dynamic pandemic: 'Woke up early this morning . . . I lay for a while, wondering what was different . . . Then it occu[r]red to me: in all the time I had lain there I had not heard a single car . . . I wonder if it was that unprecedented silence that woke me, the absence of the rumble of normality.'[61] Some respondents seemed to struggle with their desire to create entries which focused upon themselves: 'I debated whether or not to write this. I'm feeling pretty self-involved right now'.[62] Despite this, *#RecordCovid19* is

---

58 [*#RecordCovid19*–28] Oxford, Teacher, 59, http://kristopherlovell.com/2020/04/25/record-covid19-28-oxford-teacher-59/, accessed 14 April 2023.

59 [*#RecordCovid19*–85] Cambridgeshire, Content Writer, Female, 35, http://kristopherlovell.com/2020/10/05/recordcovid19-85-cambridgeshire-content-writer-female-35/.

60 [*#RecordCovid19*–7] UK, Writer, Male 18+, http://kristopherlovell.com/2020/04/14/record-covid-19-7-uk-writer-male-18/.

61 [*#RecordCovid19*–9] Bridgnorth, Bar Manager, Male, 25, http://kristopherlovell.com/2020/04/16/record-covid19-9-bridgnorth-bar-manager-male-25/.

62 [*#RecordCovid19*–15] Wales, Engineer, Female, 30, http://kristopherlovell.com/2020/04/21/record-covid-19-15-wales-engineer-female-30/.

practically defined by autobiographical reflections. 'I'm so tired', one respondent wrote, '[m]y grief has been cyclical. Sometimes I'm fine, sometimes I'm happy, sometimes I'm devastated, sometimes I'm guilty, sometimes I'm empty. Past trauma has complicated things. I've been backsliding. I'd worked so hard. I'd gotten so much healing done. I'd gotten so much growing done. How did so much slip away so fast?'[63] This autobiographical impulse is a key strength of this source-base. Early entries to *#RecordCovid19* are candid and, in many cases, deeply personal in nature. 'I have struggled with homeworking', wrote one London-based respondent, 'I've realised that my tone became more clipped and short and frustrated over the last month, and I think it's made people afraid to talk to me, because it[']s clear I'm very stressed and may not be coping well. But with no one asking me for help, or a second opinion, I just feel more alone. I'm also paranoid, and started thinking maybe they just think I'm too stupid to ask questions of.'[64]

In early entries, the self is frequently centred within an uncertain context which, in turn, problematized assumed truths about the individual. 'I feel like I'm in a bad dream', wrote one respondent.[65] Another wrote of the 'despondency' created by the coming of lockdown and 'an ever-present lowness that nothing could alleviate for long'.[66] In other words, early entries captured and underlined the existential challenges posed by the lockdown experience; what do assumed truths about one's self mean when assumed truths about one's context are obliterated? That question hangs over so many of *#RecordCovid19*'s early entries. 'I have nothing but time', wrote one respondent, '[a]nd time is such an intangible, nebulous thing, that sometimes it feels as though I have nothing at all.'[67] Over time, however, the tone of many entries began to shift, something which likely reflected changes occurring within (and to) its respondents. The deeply personal nature of many early submission became more anomalous with abstract, metaphysical concerns appearing less frequently: 'I'm much better psychologically'.[68] Over time, respondents engaged in fewer self-critical reappraisals. To be sure, entries throughout 2020 contained significant evidence of

---

63 [*#RecordCovid19*–25] Berlin, Student, Genderqueer, 25, http://kristopherlovell.com/2020/04/24/record-covid19-25-berlin-student-genderqueer-25/.

64 [*#RecordCovid19*–16] London, Civil Servant, Female, 25, http://kristopherlovell.com/2020/04/21/record-covid-19-16-london-female-25-civil-servant/.

65 [*#RecordCovid19*–1] Croydon, Civil Servant, Female, 25, http://kristopherlovell.com/2020/04/12/record-covid-19-1-croydon-civil-servant-female-25/, accessed 14 April 2023.

66 [*#RecordCovid19*–3] Lincoln, Stage Manager, Female, 29. http://kristopherlovell.com/2020/04/12/record-covid-19-3-lincoln-stage-manager-female-29/, accessed 14 April 2023.

67 [*#RecordCovid19*–18] Wales, Writer, Female, 27, http://kristopherlovell.com/2020/04/23/record-covid-19-18-wales-writer-female-27/, accessed 14 April 2023.

68 [*#RecordCovid19*–38] Turkey, Student, Female, 18, http://kristopherlovell.com/2020/04/28/record-covid19-37-turkey-student-female-18/, accessed 14 April 2023.

emotional strain, but there was also an increasing focus on the external, rather than the internal world. In particular, politicians came to occupy an ever-larger amount of the respondents' attention. 'Boris Johnson has just talked about easing the lockdown measures in England', wrote one respondent, 'so that more workers (read: minimum-wage workers) can go back to work, even though we're clearly not even slightly out of the woods'.[69] As lockdown-era scandals mounted in the UK, so too did anger towards external actors within the source-base: '[Boris] Johnson has chosen to defend the potentially illegal and dangerous actions of an individual [Dominic Cummings- with whom he has close personal and professional ties in a blatant, offensive act of nepotism. This cannot be allowed to stand'.[70] 'The English government', wrote another, 'are in [an] absolute shambles, with one foul controversy after another, and Boris Johnson – idiot at large – feels like opening schools in the middle of a pandemic is a great idea to return to normalcy.'[71]

There remains, however, the issue of audience which problematizes the autobiographical nature of these accounts. Respondents to this project were not publishing social media status updates on a whim for an audience of friends, family, and acquaintances. They had time to consider their contributions and to reflect upon what they wished to commit to the record; and who would see it. As a consequence, *#RecordCovid19* captures a very specific type of pandemic-era reflection – one which likely anticipated some expectation on the part of a perceived, albeit anonymous, audience. Many early entries, particularly the most personal in nature, provided insights that are, in the context of the source-base as a whole, remarkably revealing. It is possible that the candid nature of some entries reflected a need to make personal connections in a time when socialisation had been banned. It is also possible that respondents were engaged in a type of memorialising process, capturing something essentially honest about themselves in a time when one's wellbeing and safety (and therefore, future existence) seemed to be in acute danger. As respondents adjusted to lockdown, however, they seem to have become less inclined to engage in such processes and, as a consequence, came to focus increasingly on external factors or limited internal reflection. Whilst the presence of an audience, and the respondents' relationship to it, add additional layers of problematizing complexity to these sources, so too do they reveal interesting possibilities about how

---

69 [*#RecordCovid19–51*] Suffolk, England, Post-Graduate Student, Female, 22, http://kristopherlovell. com/2020/05/11/recordcovid19-51-suffolk-england-postgrad-student-female-22/, accessed 14 April 2023.
70 [*#RecordCovid19–57*] Wales, Writer, Female, 28, http://kristopherlovell.com/2020/05/26/record covid19-57-wales-writer-female-28/, accessed 14 April 2023.
71 [*#RecordCovid19–61*] East Yorkshire, University Student, Female, 26, http://kristopherlovell.com/ 2020/05/26/recordcovid19-61-east-yorkshire-university-student-female-26/, accessed 14 April 2023.

individuals coped with the unprecedented. These are tantalising avenues for future researchers to consider.

As the pandemic progressed, reassessment became increasingly common within submissions: '[t]rying to unravel how all of this happened so quickly is perhaps the hardest part'.[72] If early entries were more likely to describe in-the-moment sensations, feelings, and fears, then later entries became spaces in which assessment and analysis were more common with respondents showing increased levels of interest in ascribing meaning to recent events. 'Looking back at the time I posted my first entry', wrote one, 'I remember the feeling of pessimism'.[73] The autobiographical process was thus captured *in motu*. This allows researchers consulting *#RecordCovid19* to observe the process of coping and understanding which paralleled the course of the pandemic. The impulse to create autobiographical accounts, whilst certainly creating some problematizing issues for these sources, also creates distinct opportunities for understanding internal change over the course of the pandemic.

Closure

Lockdown cannot be easily disentangled from the process of storytelling. Its unprecedented nature created a series of existential crises for many of those who experienced it and, lacking lived experience which could inform their understanding of events, they looked to stories for answers and escape. Socially isolated and frequently scared, individuals sought solace in the tales they consumed, and the stories they themselves were creating. Prior entertainment products provided context. Fantastic tales provided perspective, allowing for a process of narrative relativism that was, for many, a vital part of the pandemic's lived experience. When the world seemed it's most unreal, melodramatic stories about survival and global disasters took on a new socio-cultural function. But it was escapist-fare that people seemed to need the most. Intergalactic bounty hunters, superheroes, and rogue zookeepers seized the zeitgeist, even as individuals sought to support themselves, their family, and their peers through the unfolding crisis. Narratives came to serve multiple functions; escape, support, and perspective.

---

72 [*#RecordCovid19*–105] Birmingham, UK, Student, Male, 21, http://kristopherlovell.com/2020/12/23/recordcovid19-105-birmingham-united-kingdom-male-21-student/, accessed 14 April 2023.

73 [*#RecordCovid19*–112] Turkey, Student, Female, 20, http://kristopherlovell.com/2021/01/31/recordcovid19-112-turkey-student-female-20/, accessed 14 April 2023.

#RecordCovid19 occurred within this context, providing another form of narrative escapism. Rather than consuming stories, its respondents were provided with an opportunity to become active participants in the creative process. It provided a space in which individuals could memorialise or record new feelings and thoughts; reach out from socially isolated spaces; and explore the complex emotions that the pandemic had created. Within *#RecordCovid19*, the importance of narrative appears in multiple ways, from direct references to disaster movies, to the stories that respondents themselves were telling. Individuals related to narratives, and they created them. Parents told children stories; friends shared experiences; and families worked together to place their pandemic-era experiences into context. In a series of evolving autobiographical accounts, respondents demonstrated that consumption and creation were key aspects of the lockdown era. Stories were not told arbitrarily. Story had an important function to serve. Autobiographical accounts steeped in narrative relativism may not communicate the precise factual reality of the pandemic, but they do capture some of the nuance that helped to define so many lived experiences during the lockdown-era.

References

Abrams, Lynn. Oral History Theory. London and New York: Routledge, 2016.

Assmann, Jan. 'Collective Memory and Cultural Identity.' New German Critique 65 (1995): 125–133.

Ball, Philip and Amy Maxmen. 'The Epic Battle against Coronavirus Misinformation and Conspiracy Theories.' Nature, May 27, 2020. https://www.nature.com/articles/d41586-020-01452-z. Accessed 8 February 2023.

Bat, Martina. 'Coronavirus Action Plan: How Boris Johnson Said "He is Inspired by Mayor from Jaws"' The Independent, 13 March 2020. https://www.express.co.uk/news/uk/1254769/coronavirus-uk-news-cases-deaths-schools-boris-johnson-strategy-jaws-major-spt. Accessed 8 February 2023.

Berryman, Charles. 'Critical Mirrors: Theories of Autobiography.' Mosaic: An Interdisciplinary Critical Journal 32 (1999): 71–84.

Bonnet, Alma Pierre. 'The "Churchill Factor" and its Influence on the Brexit Debate: Defining the Churchill Myth.' Observatoire de la Société Britannique 25 (2020):65–86.

Bornat, Joanna. 'Oral History and Remembering' in Research Methods for Memory Studies, edited by Emily Keightley and Michael Pickering, 29–42. Edinburgh: Edinburgh University Press, 2013.

Brundage, W. Fitzhugh. 'Commemoration and Conflict: Forgetting and Remembering the Civil War' The Georgia Historical Quarterly 82 (1998): 559–574.

Campbell, Joseph. The Hero with a Thousand Faces, 3rd edition. New York: Pantheon Books, 1949; reprint, Novato: New World Library, 2008.

Confino, Alon. 'Collective Memory and Cultural History: Problems of Method.' The American Historical Review 102 (1997): 1386–1403.

Dunn, Katherine. 'To Tackle Coronavirus, Brits are Appealing to an Age-Old Rallying Cry: "Blitz Spirit".' Fortune, 6 March 2020. https://fortune.com/2020/03/06/coronavirus-brexit-blitz-spirit. Accessed 8 February 2023.

Faulkenbury, Evan. '"A Problem of Visibility": Remembering and Forgetting the Civil War in Cortland, New York.' The Public Historian 41 (2019): 83–99.

Fear, David. 'How "Contagion" Suddenly Became the Most Urgent Movie of 2020.' Rolling Stone, 13 March 2020. https://www.rollingstone.com/movies/movie-features/contagion-most-urgent-movie-of-2020-964532. Accessed 8 February 2023.

Feder, Gene., Ana Flavia, Lucas d'Oliveira, Poonam Risha and Medina Johnson. 'Domestic Violence during the Pandemic.' BMJ 372 (2021): n722. https://doi.org/10.1136/bmj.n722

Flood, Alison. 'UK Book Sales Soared in 2020 Despite Pandemic.' The Guardian, 27 April 2020. https://www.theguardian.com/books/2021/apr/27/uk-book-sales-soared-in-2020-despite-pandemic. Accessed 8 February 2023.

Grant, Kirsty. 'Covid: Lessons I Learned from Lockdowns in 2020.' BBC News, 5 January 2021. https://www.bbc.co.uk/news/newsbeat-54791791. Accessed 8 February 2023.

Harrison, Rebecca. 'The Mandalorian Season 2 Seeks Hope in a Bruised and Battered Galaxy.' BFI, December 21, 2020. https://www.bfi.org.uk/sight-and-sound/reviews/mandalorian-season-2-star-wars-spin-off-disney-grogu-din-djarin. Accessed 8 February 2023.

Heritage, Stuart. 'Boris Johnson's Hero is the Mayor Who Kept the Beaches Open in Jaws. That's Fine By Me.' The Guardian, March 13, 2020. https://www.theguardian.com/film/2020/mar/13/boris-johnson-coronavirus-hero-mayor-larry-vaughn-jaws. Accessed 8 February 2023.

Hersko, Tyler. '"The Mandalorian" Review: Season 2 Ends with a Noisy, Mindless Slaughter.' IndieWire, December 18, 2020. https://www.indiewire.com/2020/12/the-mandalorian-review-season-2-finale-1234605624. Accessed 8 February 2023.

Hetata, Sherif. 'The Self and Autobiography' PMLA 118 (2003): 123–125.

Kansteiner, Wulf. 'Finding Meaning in Memory: A Methodological Critique of Collective Memory Studies.' History and Theory 41 (2002): 179–197.

Katz, Brandon. 'The 10 Most Watched Movies on Netflix During Lockdown.' The Observer, April 21, 2020. https://observer.com/2020/04/netflix-ratings-most-watched-movies-what-to-stream-covid-19. Accessed 8 February 2023.

Kelsey, Darren. 'The Myth of the "Blitz Spirit" in British Newspaper Responses to the July 7th Bombings.' Social Semiotics 23 (2013): 83–99.

Kruegar, Kori L. and Forest, Amanda L. 'Communicating Commitment: A Relationship-Protection Account of Dyadic Displays on Social Media.' Personality and Social Psychology Bulletin 46 (2020): 1059–1073.

Mangan, Dan. 'Trump Blames China for Coronavirus Pandemic: "The World is paying a Very Big Price for What They Did.' CNBC, March 19, 2020. https://www.cnbc.com/2020/03/19/coronavirus-outbreak-trump-blames-china-for-virus-again.html. Accessed 8 February 2023.

Mendelson, Scott. 'Box Office: "Soul" Nabs $6M in China as "Croods 2" Nears $100M Global.' Forbes, December 27, 2020. https://www.forbes.com/sites/scottmendelson/2021/12/27/box-office-soul-nabs-6m-in-china-as-croods-2-nears-100m-global/?sh=7e95904c327a. Accessed 8 February 2023.

Nicholas, Siân. 'History, Revisionism, and Television Drama: Foyle's War and the "Myth of 1940".' Media History 13 (2007): 203–219.

Nicholson, Rebecca. 'Insane, Intoxicating Tiger King is Perfect Lockdown TV.' The Guardian, April 4, 2020. https://www.theguardian.com/commentisfree/2020/apr/04/insane-intoxicating-tale-of-big-cats-is-perfect-lockdown-tv-tiger-watch-james-mcavoy-greta-gerwig. Accessed 8 February 2023.

Oppenheim, Maya. 'Divorce Enquiries to Legal Firms Soar by 95% in Pandemic with Women Driving Surge in Interest.' The Independent, May 8, 2021. https://www.independent.co.uk/news/uk/home-news/divorce-inquiries-rise-pandemic-women-b1843359.html. Accessed 8 February 2023.

Overy, Richard. 'Why the Cruel Myth of the "Blitz Spirit" is No Model for How to Fight Coronavirus.' The Guardian, March 19th, 2020. https://www.theguardian.com/commentisfree/2020/mar/19/myth-blitz-spirit-model-coronavirus. Accessed 8 February 2023.

Palm, Christopher and Shaw, Lucas. '"Tiger King" Documentary a Netflix Hit in Coronavirus Lockdown.' Bloomberg, April 8, 2020. https://www.bloomberg.com/news/articles/2020-04-08/netflix-s-quirky-tiger-king-becomes-breakout-pandemic-hit. Accessed 8 February 2023.

Palmer, Anthony and Champlin, T.S. Champlin. 'Self-Deception: A Problem about Autobiography' Proceedings of the Aristotelian Society, Supplementary 53 (1979): 61–94.

Perez, Matt. 'U.S. Video Game Sales Set Record Second Quarter, Spurred by Pandemic.' Forbes, August 10, 2020. https://www.forbes.com/sites/mattperez/2020/08/10/video-games-set-record-second-quarter-spurred-by-pandemic-sales/?sh=5aa346ef6f4e. Accessed 8 February 2023.

Prudom, Laura. 'The Mandalorian: Season 2 Review.' IGN, December 23rd, 2020: https://www.ign.com/articles/the-mandalorian-season-2-review. Accessed 8 February 2023.

Radstone, Susannah and Schwarz, Bill. Memory: Histories, Theories Debates. New York: Fordham University Press, 2010.

Ritchie, Donald A. Doing Oral History. Oxford: Oxford University Press, 2015.

Rosenberg, Alex. How History Gets Things Wrong: The Neuroscience of Our Addiction to Stories. Cambridge: MIT Press, 2018.

Ryan, Patrick. 'The Storyteller in Context: Storyteller Identity and Storytelling Experience' Storytelling, Self, Society 4 (2008): 64–87.

Sprinker, Michael. 'Fictions of the Self: The End of Autobiography' in Autobiography: Essays Theoretical and Critical, edited by James Olney, 321–342. Princeton: Princeton University Press, 1980.

Stewart, Heather. 'Cummings Brought to Life What Many Already Knew About Johnson's Failures.' The Guardian, May 26, 2021. https://www.theguardian.com/politics/2021/may/26/cummings-brought-to-life-what-many-already-knew-about-johnsons-failures. Accessed 8 February 2023.

Thomson, Alistair. 'Oral History and Community History in Britain: Personal and Critical Reflections on Twenty-Five Years of Continuity and Change' Oral History 36 (2008): 95–104.

Thomson, Paul. The Voice of the Past: Oral History. Oxford: Oxford University Press, 1988.

Trower, Shelley. 'Auto/Biographical Oral Histories, from "Oral Memories" to "The Life of Nate Shaw"' Oral History 45 (2017): 43–45.

Woodcock, Andrew. '"Disastrous" Mistakes Caused Tens of Thousands of Unnecessary Deaths from Covid, says Dominic Cummings.' The Independent, 26 May 2021. https://www.independent.co.uk/news/uk/politics/dominic-cummings-covid-boris-johnson-b1854048.html. Accessed 8 February 2023.

Wyatt, Tim. 'Boris Johnson Has History of Comparing Himself to Jaws' Reckless Mayor Who Kept Beaches Open.' The Independent, 27 April 2021. https://www.independent.co.uk/news/uk/politics/boris-johnson-jaws-mayor-beach-b1838049.html. Accessed 8 February 2023.

'Covid-19 & Me': https://libguides.princeton.edu/c.php?g=937179&p=7407469

Covid-19 Oral History Project': https://covid-19archive.org

Coronavirus: Trump Stands by China Lab Origin Theory for Virus.' BBC News, 1 May 2020. https://www.bbc.co.uk/news/world-us-canada-52496098. Accessed 8 February 2023.

Covid: Boris Johnson's "Bodies Pile High" Comments Prompt Criticism.' BBC News, 26 April 2021. https://www.bbc.co.uk/news/uk-politics-56890714. Accessed 8 February 2023.

Spirit of the Blitz.' The Economist, 21 March 2020. https://www.economist.com/britain/2020/03/21/spirit-of-the-blitz. Accessed 8 February 2023.

The Irish COVID-19 Oral History Project': https://covid19oralhistory.ie.

TV Watching and Online Streaming Surge during Lockdown.' BBC News, 5 August 2020. https://www.bbc.co.uk/news/entertainment-arts-53637305. Accessed 8 February 2023.

Arddun Arwyn
Chapter Eight
Crisis and Storytelling: Learning Lessons from the Past

The *#RecordCovid19* project set out to capture the responses to and narratives of crisis by everyday people and is an important repository of stories about an unfolding crisis. Critically understanding narratives of crisis told by individuals and societies is more significant than one might think. They directly impact how we move forward from and learn from difficult times. This chapter addresses exactly that. It takes two seemingly different crises, Covid-19 pandemic and the expulsion of Germans after World War Two and demonstrates that there are distinct patterns in the stories constructed about both events. Such patterns of narration are also common across many crises and are noteworthy because the stories we tell about events impact political and policy responses as well as public opinion. Using the work of Matthew W. Seeger and Timothy L. Sellnow to categorise stories of times of crisis, the chapter outlines how both examples provide lessons for the critical understanding crises narratives and the real-world impact of such stories on our perception and actions.

To understand the construction of crisis narratives Matthew W. Seeger and Timothy L. Sellnow developed a typology to categorise the representation of crisis in the modern world. Their research has demonstrated that: by looking at narratives of different crises we can categorise narratives into distinct types: narratives of blame, victimhood, heroism, renewal and memorialisation (each of these will be explored in detail in each section).[1] Using this typology, the chapter explores narratives of Covid-19 and the flight and expulsion of Germans and how both crises correspond to this typology. Although these crises are different in nature (one a pandemic and the other a refugee crisis) we can nevertheless find similarities in the narratives that have been constructed about them. This is significant as the way we speak about crisis has a direct impact on how we act in the real world, on political action and policy and on the ways, we move forward and learn from the past. They also help us better appreciate how humans make sense of difficult times. By unpicking these two sets of crisis narratives and understanding their common features across time and cultures, we can become more critical about

---

[1] Matthew W. Seeger and Timothy L. Sellnow, *Narratives of Crisis. Telling Stories of Ruin and Renewal* (Stanford: Stanford University Press, 2016), 13–14.

https://doi.org/10.1515/9783110731002-009

information and how it is shared. Thus, working towards mitigating the damage of divisive and harmful myths and conspiracies that emerge from times of crisis, poisoning our future as well as our perception of the past.

This chapter will address three main questions: How do the narratives of German expellees and the Covid-19 pandemic relate to Seeger and Sellnow's taxonomy? What are the main features of these crisis narratives? And, finally, what can we learn from narratives of crisis? First the chapter will introduce the German expellees and their history and background. Then, it will address the narratives of Germans expelled from Eastern Europe and Covid–19 in relation to the typology of narratives of crisis, beginning with blame, then moving onto victims, heroes, renewal and finally memorialisation.

Background – Who Are the German Expellees?

Until the end of the Second World War Germans had lived in communities scattered across Eastern Europe for centuries. Some lived in regions of Germany that were lost due to border changes and others lived as ethnic minorities within other states. As a result of the genocidal and expansionist war undertaken by the Nazis up to twelve million Germans living in Eastern Europe were displaced. The displacement of Germans in the period 1945–48 came in numerous forms. A number were relocated by the Nazis during the war to colonize occupied Poland; others left their homes as refugees fleeing the Soviet invasion and the rest were expelled from countries, such as Poland and Czechoslovakia, where they had lived as ethnic minorities.[2] This chapter will focus on the narratives that stem from one former German region, East Prussia.

The history of German settlement in East Prussia began with the Teutonic Knights in the thirteenth century who conquered the area and Christianised its Baltic population. It then became a significant territory within the Kingdom of Prussia before being separated from the rest of Germany by the Polish Corridor after the First World War.[3] In the final elections of the Weimar Republic East

---

2 For an excellent overview of the history of the expulsions see: R. M. Douglas, *Orderly and Humane: The Expulsion of the Germans after the Second World War* (New Haven: Yale University Press, 2012).

3 Two histories of East Prussia have been published recently: Andreas Kossert, *Ostpreußen: Geschichte und Mythos*, 3rd edn. (Munich: Pantheon, 2009) and Hermann Pölking, *Ostpreußen: Biographie einer Provinz* (Berlin: Bebra, 2011). There is no English language history of East Prussia but Christopher Clarke's *The Iron Kingdom. The Rise and Downfall of Prussia, 1600–1947* (London: Penguin, 2006) provides an excellent general history of Prussia.

Prussia returned some of the largest returns for the NSDAP. During the Third Reich the province was largely supportive of the regime and put up no significant resistance to the crimes committed in its name such as deportation of Jews and the use of forced labour. In 1945, the Soviet Red Army invaded and significant numbers of East Prussia's 2.5 million inhabitants fled westward.[4] Those who were left behind joined the other circa twelve million Germans who were expelled from Eastern Europe during the period 1945–1948.[5] After the war East Prussia was divided between Russia (then USSR) and Poland as it remains today. Those Germans displaced from East Prussia, and other areas, were resettled across the four Zones of Occupation which later became East (GDR) and West Germany (FRG) in 1949.[6] The experiences of fleeing, expulsion and resettlement were highly traumatic and amounted to a prolonged crisis that plays a central role in the identities and memories of East Prussians to this day. Here we will focus on the displaced Germans who settled in West Germany and who came to be known as expellees.[7]

Blame

The first category in Seeger and Sellnow's taxonomy is blame. Attributing blame is a central tenet of narratives of crisis as it provides meaning to painful and seemingly uncontrollable events. Seeger and Sellnow argue that blame narratives tend to take up much space and play out publicly. Typically, the accuser puts forward narratives

---

4 Numbers are notoriously difficult to obtain and should be treated with caution as they have been politicised by expellee organisations. See Kossert, *Ostpreußen*, 330.

5 Again, here numbers are very unreliable. There were circa 140,000 German in the Northern Part of East Prussia in September 1945 according to a Soviet census, Ruth Kibelka, *Ostpreußens Schicksalsjahre 1944–1945* (Berlin, Edition Berolina, 2016), 46. Not all ethnic Germans or ethnically diverse German speakers (identities are very complex in these regions) were expelled after the war. Some stayed in Eastern Europe and migrated later. See Richard Blanke, *"Polish-Speaking Germans?" Language and National Identity Among the Masurians* (Cologne: Bohlau, 2001) and David W. Gerlach, *The Economy of Ethnic Cleansing: The Transformation of the German-Czech borderlands after World War II* (Cambridge, Cambridge University Press, 2017).

6 Displaced Germans were treated differently depending on where they lived in divided Germany. In East Germany the GDR their victimhood as a result of the close relationship between the state and the USSR. For further information on displaced Germans in East Germany see Ian Connor, *Refugees and Expellees in post–war* Germany (Manchester: Manchester University Press, 2007), 197–234 and Michael Schwarz, 'Vertriebene in doppelten Deutschland,' *Vierteljahrshefte für Zeitgeschichte* 56:1 (2008): 101–150.

7 This chapter will draw on a range of sources by German expellees from individual accounts in oral histories, autobiographical texts, periodicals and museums.

with the aim of achieving accountability for the crisis through public scorn. Competing narratives often develop in relation to this type, as accusers attempt to redress the balance, avoid responsibility, and claims of restitution.[8] These functions can also be seen in the blame narratives relating to both expellees and the Covid-19 crisis.

In the narratives of expellees, the invading Red Army is painted as the principal culprits. Within these narratives of blame little or no reflection is given to the role of German civilians in the regime and its crimes. Deeply held myths and oversimplified stereotypes blame one or two figures, obscuring the support given by German civilians to the war and regime, which is problematic given the regime's involvement in the biggest genocide in history.[9] Concurrently, shared figures of blame are powerful integrative tools as the community comes together in solidarity through feelings of injustice. Therefore, on one hand blame is used to deflect responsibility and on the other it has become a source of cohesion for the group.

It is understandable why much of the blame for German suffering is placed on the Red Army by expellees. The full invasion of East Prussia began in January 1945 and the civilians' experience of it was brutal.[10] Acts committed against civilians included violence, death, sexual violence and plunder.[11] Civilians were not given permission to flee until the last minute, meaning they often came into direct contact with fighting. The roads, trains and ships evacuating East Prussians were often utterly chaotic and dangerous. It was also winter with temperatures plummeting to minus thirty degrees. The narratives of flight are harrowing and convey extreme suffering where women, children and the elderly were the main victims.

---

8 Seeger & Sellnow, *Narratives*, 64.

9 This is a commonly held view among scholars working on expellees. See Andrew Demshuk, *The Lost German East: Forced Migration and the Politics of Memory, 1945–1970* (Cambridge: Cambridge University Press, 2012), 10; Alfred Lehmann, *Im Fremden ungewollt zu haus: Flüchtlinge und Vertriebene in Westdeutschland, 1945–1990* (Munich: C.H.Beck, 1991), 195–199.

10 East Prussia was under military threat from 1944 onwards. Some areas were invaded and occupied beginning in summer and autumn 1944. The main invasion did not however, begin until the 12th of January 1945. Bastian Willems provides a comprehensive account of the military situation in Bastian Wilems, *Violence in Defeat* (Cambridge: Cambridge University Press, 2021).

11 The West German government commissioned historians to collect accounts by civilians of their experiences of flight and expulsion in which their mistreatment is documented. These were edited and published as the multi-volume: Theodor Schieder, ed., *Dokumentation der Vertreibung der Deutschen aus Ost–Mitteleuropa* (Bonn, Bundesministerium für Vertriebene, 1954–1961). An English language version was also produced: Theodor Schieder, ed., *Documents on the expulsion of the Germans from Eastern-Central-Europe*: A selection and translation from *Dokumentation der Vertreibung der Deutschen aus Ost–Mitteleuropa*, Bd. 1, 1–2; Bd 2; Bd. 4, 1–2 (Bonn, Bundesministerium für Vertriebene, 1954–1961).

Most expellee narratives of the Red Army are racist and coloured by Nazi and older stereotypes.[12] Red Army soldiers are often portrayed as either a violent, 'bestial' and 'Asiatic hoard' that swept over East Prussia in a wave of wonton violence and destruction or as simple and incompetent fools with a fondness for small children.[13] There are some exceptions, but they largely confirm the rule. Within these portrayals of misery there is a tendency to forget the role of the German-led war in the invasion. Little mind is paid to the Holocaust and various crimes committed by the German forces during their invasion and occupation of Eastern Europe and the USSR. Therefore, the narratives tend to portray the invasion as a sudden and unexpected attack on an innocent people. This focus on narratives of blame results in little space for reflecting on individuals' role in the causes of these catastrophic events.

Narratives of blame can also be recognised in the Covid-19 crisis. Already in the opening weeks of the Covid-19 blame was being attributed to all kinds of people and objects, from the lowly bat and the protected pangolin to the entire Chinese nation. These narratives of blame that emerged in those early frightening and confusing times had real and very dangerous consequences. East Asian of varying ethnicities living in the USA and the UK experienced hate crimes and racisim.[14] Bats were attacked and killed globally. In the early days of the pandemic some blamed new technologies for the spread of the virus and 5G mobile phone towers were targeted and burnt down by those who feared their role in the virus.[15] These wild narratives that circulated at a time when mass uncertainty spanned the globe and

---

12 This has been studied comprehensively in the following books: Michael Burleigh, *Germany Turns Eastwards: A Study of Ostforschung in the Third Reich* (London: Pan, 2002); Vejas Gabriel Liulevicius, *The German Myth of the East: 1800 to the Present* (Oxford: Oxford University Press USA, 2011); Robert L. Nelson, ed., *Germans, Poland, and Colonial Expansion to the East: 1850 Through the Present* (Basingstoke; New York: Palgrave Macmillan, 2014).

13 Lehmann, *Im Fremden*, 196; Norman Naimark, *The Russians in Germany: A History of the Soviet Zone of Occupation, 1945–1949* (Harvard: Harvard University Press, 1995), 82–83.

14 Angela R. Gover, Shannon B. Harper and Lynn Langton, "Anti-Asian Hate Crime During the COVID-19 Pandemic: Exploring the Reproduction of Inequality," *American Journal of Criminal Justice* 45 (2020): 647–667, 649; Jamie Grierson, "Anti-Asian Hate Crimes Up 21% In UK During Coronavirus Crisis," *The Guardian*, 13 May 2020, https://www.theguardian.com/world/2020/may/13/anti-asian-hate-crimes-up-21-in-uk-during-coronavirus-crisis accessed 28 June 2022; Jason Bittel, "Experts Urge People All Over the World to Stop Killing Bats out of Fear of Coronavirus," *Natural Resources Defense Council*, https://www.nrdc.org/stories/experts-urge-people-all-over-world-stop-killing-bats-out-fears-coronavirus, accessed 28 June 2022.

15 Adam Satariano and Davey Alba, 'Burning Cell Towers, Out of Baseless Fear They Spread the Virus,' *New York Times*, 10 April 2020, https://www.nytimes.com/2020/04/10/technology/coronavirus-5g-uk.html, accessed 20 June 2022.

people sought understanding and meaning. These examples demonstrate clearly how narratives of blame can fuel violence and hatred in times of crisis.

Moving beyond the opening weeks of the crisis a general sense of mismanagement prevailed in the UK resulting in narratives of blame developing around the government and its leader Boris Johnson. The perception that the UK government hesitated in implementing a lockdown combined with a high case and death rate in the spring of 2020 resulted in UK leaders being criticised by some media outlets.[16] Blame compounded with a series of outrages when it emerged that the Prime Minister's right hand man Dominic Cummings had broken the strict first 2020 lockdown rules to visit his parents on two occasions.[17] This resulted in further mistrust of the government and general outrage among the population. Fast forward the tape to spring 2022 when details of numerous parties being held throughout the pandemic, including during the strict periods of lockdown, emerged. As part of the 'Partygate Scandal' highly damaging images of a cheese and wine party where top government officials and politicians, including the Prime Minister, were in attendance were leaked.[18] The outrage among MPs resulted in a vote of no-confidence against the PM, which he narrowly won. Despite this win the harm to his reputation was severe and he was pushed to resign by July 2022 with a series of scandals and accusations of incompetence hanging over him.[19] The narrative of blame for the crisis shifted from accounting for its actual cause to accusations against the Conservative government of corruption and mismanagement.

Narratives of blame clearly shape our perception and understandings of crisis. Although the two crises under consideration were very different in nature there are similar patterns in how people narrate blame. In both cases racism and damaging stereotypes influenced the attribution of blame to a perceived racial 'other'. These perceptions were harmful in both cases with many expellees continuing to

---

16 Heather Stewart and Ian Sample, "Coronavirus: enforcing UK lockdown one week earlier 'could have saved 20,000 lives,' *The Guardian*, 11 June 2020, https://www.theguardian.com/world/2020/jun/10/uk-coronavirus-lockdown-20000-lives-boris-johnson-neil-ferguson accessed 28 June 2022; Jonathon Calvert, George Arbuthnott and Jonathan Leake, 'Coronavirus: 38 Days When Britain Sleepwalked Into Disaster,' *The Times*, 19 April 2020, https://www.thetimes.co.uk/article/coronavirus-38-days-when-britain-sleepwalked-into-disaster-hq3b9tlgh, accessed 28 June 2022.

17 Joe Pike, "Coronavirus: Dominic Cummings Made Second Trip To Durham During Lockdown," *Sky News*, https://news.sky.com/story/coronavirus-dominic-cummings-made-second-trip-to-durham-during-lockdown-reports-11993660, accessed 28 June 2022.

18 Anon., "Partygate: A Timeline of Lockdown Gatherings," *BBC News*, accessed 28 June 2020 https://www.bbc.com/news/uk-politics-59952395, accessed 14 April 2023.

19 Owen Amos, "Boris Johnson Resigns: Five Things That Led To The PM's Downfall," *BBC News*, 7 July 2022, https://www.bbc.com/news/uk-politics–62070422, accessed 14 April 2023.

hold racist views of Russians and East Asians being singled out for prejudice and attack since the beginning of the pandemic. In both cases blame has garnered solidarity which has contributed to the shaping of political views and action. The lesson to be learnt here is that blame narratives are powerful and can fuel deep emotional responses which can result in the hardening of political views. By learning to understand how these narratives are formed and shared we can better educate people on how to respond to them critically and with some rationality.

Victims

Victim narratives are also some of the most powerful to emerge from crises. Seeger and Seelow note that they are very common and give a human face to catastrophe. Beyond personification they also tend to cast victims as morally innocent, often leading to one sided representations. They also are important in influencing public opinion as they shape perceptions of empathy and blame.[20] As will be demonstrated, they also serve as a powerful political tool as they are a source of identity, communal solidarity and for calls for political action and restitution. As was the case with German expellees who have drawn deeply on victim narratives to leverage political and financial support. In the Covid-19 crisis, victim narratives have played an important role in drawing attention to governmental policy failures in the UK.

In expellee culture, narratives of victimhood are central to their self-perception. They had legitimately suffered during their flight from Eastern Europe and those who remained in Eastern Europe after May 1945 also underwent severe hardships, including starvation, forced labour, persecution, and violence. The deportations westwards were often horrific. Railway carriages were overfilled, the sick and elderly died where they lay – there were even reports of a pregnant woman miscarrying and her blood freezing her to the carriage floor.[21] Their resettlement across Germany was traumatic. The country was destroyed by war and resources were scarce. Therefore, millions of incoming expellees were not welcomed by the struggling German population, who were forced by the Allies to take in the displaced. There were also distinct regional differences between Germans, with dialects, confession and culture varying and so many expellees experienced prejudice and

---

20 Seeger & Sellnow, *Narratives*, 98–99.
21 Andreas Kossert, *Kalte Heimat: Die Geschichte der deutschen Vertriebenen nach 1945* (Munich: Pantheon Verlag, 2009), 51.

discrimination.[22] These narratives are central to individual recollections as well as a collective sense of identity propagated by organisations representing expellees. Victim narratives have been a powerful unifying force among expellees. However, as in the case of narratives of blame, expellees have tended to focus on their own victimhood without reflecting on the crimes of Nazism and their own actions in the cause of their suffering.[23]

The relationship between narratives of victimhood and political action is very clear in the case of the expellees. The West German government's categorisation of expellees as German victims of the Second World War resulted in them being compensated materially, in political influence and an investment in the preservation of their regional cultures.[24] To understand these actions we must first discuss the context of the 1950s. West Germany's first post-war government was deeply pro-Western and anti-Communist. This was the height of the Cold War and West Germany's Chancellor Konrad Adenauer was steering the country towards western integration and away from the USSR and the GDR. As a result, the victimhood of the expelled Germans at the hands of either the Soviet Union or 'expeller' countries in the Soviet Bloc (i.e. Czechoslovakia and Poland) was a perfect propaganda tool against Communism.[25]

Concurrently, West Germany's relationship with the recent past also played a role in the perception of the expellees as victims. German victimhood was the predominant image of the Second World War circulating in the public realm in 1950s West Germany. Speeches by politicians, political and public discourse, as well as

---

22 Ian Connor, *Refugees and Expellees in Post–War Germany* (Manchester: Manchester University Press, 2007), 60–61; Kossert, *Kalte Heimat*, 43–71.

23 Important note: expellees and the organisations that represent them have often been criticised for a lack of introspection when expressing belonging, loss and nostalgia for the lands from which they were expelled, especially when doing so without considering the role of German aggression in the causes of the expulsions. See: Bill Niven, 'Implicit Equations in Constructions of German Suffering,' in *A Nation of Victims? Representations of German Wartime Suffering from 1945 to the Present*, ed. Helmut Schmitz, (Amsterdam: New York: Rodopi, 2007), 114–5; This theme has been extensively explored throughout: Eva Hahn and Hans Henning Hahn, *Die Vertreibung im deutschen Erinnern. Legenden, Mythos, Geschichte* (Paderborn: Verlag Ferdinand Schöningh, 2010).

24 The West German government of the 1950s prioritised the overturning of the post–1945 borders in its foreign policy towards the Eastern Bloc. Although even the Chancellor Konrad Adenauer is cited as knowing the East was lost, they did not admit this publicly and pursued an aggressive line against Eastern Communist countries. Pertti Ahonen, "Domestic Constraints on West German Ostpolitik: The Role of the Expellee Organizations in the Adenauer Era," *Central European History* 31, no. 1–2 (1998): 48, https://doi.org/10.1017/S0008938900016034.

25 The relationship between the West German government and the expellee lobby is covered in detail in Pertti Ahonen, *After the Expulsion: West Germany and Eastern Europe, 1945–1990* (Oxford; New York: Oxford University Press, 2003).

the material culture of the Federal Republic overwhelmingly contained references to German victims. Victims of Nazism, such as Jews, Eastern Europeans and the political left were, however, absent from these narratives.[26] The memory of the FRG's recent past often centred on German victimhood rather than the victims of Nazism and the Holocaust. The expellees fitted this bill nicely.[27] Victim narratives by expellees, therefore, took centre stage in the ways in which West Germans remembered the Second World War in the 1950s and the government enacted a series of initiatives to support the displaced. These included economic support to resettle, financial and political support for the 'expellee organisations' (i.e., *the League of German Expellees*) and funding to record their experiences. The powerful expellee organisations of the 1950s were able to use victim narratives to lobby for foreign policy favourable to their cause. A central tenet of West Germany's 'Eastern Policy' post-WWII was the refusal to recognise the GDR's Eastern border, the 'Order-Neisse Line', and to call for the restitution of the former German lands beyond it. The logic for this was closely related to the centrality of the narrative of victimhood propagated by the expellee organisations and taken up by the government. As recognised by Seeger and Sellnow victim narratives have powerful consequences in the real world by bringing about policy change and garnering support.[28]

During the Covid-19 crisis in the UK residents of care homes were put in danger by a series of policy failures early in the pandemic that led to preventable deaths. Since then, care home victim narratives have become an important part of the representation of the crisis. In the first weeks and months of the pandemic the British health minister Matt Hancock oversaw the release of care home residents from hospitals without routine Covid-19 testing. This compounded with insufficient safety procedures and equipment (i.e. masks and gowns) and the failure to isolate incoming patients, resulting in the virus spreading among vulnerable care home residents.[29] The narrative that unfolded highlighted the incompetence of the British

---

26 Robert G. Moeller, *War Stories: The Search for a Usable Past in the Federal Republic of Germany* (Berkely and Los Angeles: University of California Press, 2003), 12.

27 This, however, did change over time with a more 'Holocaust-cantered' memory developing in the 1960s. See Robert G. Moeller, "Sinking Ships, the Lost Heimat and Broken Taboos: Günter Grass and the Politics of Memory in Contemporary Germany," *Contemporary European History* 12:2 (2003): 159–65, https://doi.org/10.1017/S0960777303001139.

28 Seeger & Sellnow, *Narratives*, 109.

29 Reuters, "UK's Transfer of Old Patients to Care Homes in Pandemic Was Unlawful – Court," *Reuters*, 27 April 2022, https://www.reuters.com/world/uk/uks-transfer-old-patients-care-homes-pandemic-was-unlawful-court-2022-04-27/, accessed 21 June 2022; Robert Booth, "Matt Hancock "Was Warned of Covid Care Home Risk in March 2020," *The Guardian*, 9 June 2021, https://www.theguardian.com/society/2021/jun/09/matt-hancock-was-warned-of-covid-care-home-risk-in-march-2020, accessed June 21, 2022; "UK: Older people in care homes abandoned to die amid

government in safeguarding the most vulnerable. The excess deaths of 20,000 elderly in care homes became a significant Covid-19 scandal. It has also resulted in bereaved families seeking recognition through the courts system. These narratives furthered the view of the government as incompetent and uncaring in its early response, which have compounded with the narratives of blame highlighted above. The counter narrative put forward in defence by the English government was that a 'protective ring' had been placed around care homes in the early days of the pandemic and that Matt Hancock had been correct in his approach. However, a 2022 court case ruled that the discharge of patients from hospitals to care homes was illegal.[30] These debates are still ongoing at the time of writing.

Victim narratives are very important in the wake of a crisis as they bring people together and often form the basis for claims for restitution. In both cases victim narratives have been central to political and legal action. The recognition of expellees as German victims led to economic and political support from the FRG's government. In the ongoing legal action against the UK government families have coalesced around victim narratives to bring accountability and to prevent future poor management. It is interesting to note how the two examples diverge on accountability. The expellee victim narratives tend to obscure the responsibility of Germans in causing the war and thus their expulsion and in doing so avoid responsibility and accountability. Whereas in the Covid-19 victim narratives attributing accountability is central to their message. Victim narratives are interesting as they converge with narratives of blame to highlight failures and wrongdoing with the outcome of aiding societies with coming to terms with crises.

Heroes

This next group of narratives are directly related to the previous two. We have our 'baddies' or those we want to blame for crisis, then we have 'goodies' – the 'innocent victims' and then the valiant 'heroes'. Seegner and Sellow recognise three categories of heroes in crisis narratives. These were 'every day'/citizen heroes, first responder heroes and the leader hero. Versions of these archetypes are reflected in the expellee and Covid-19 narratives. In expellee narratives mothers are often represented as the

government failures during COVID-19 pandemic," Amnesty International, https://www.amnesty.org/en/latest/news/2020/10/uk-older-people-in-care-homes-abandoned-to-die-amid-government-failures-during-covid-19-pandemic/, accessed 21 June 2022.

30 Anon., "Discharging Untested Patients To Care Homes 'Unlawful,'" BBC News, 27 April 2022, https://www.bbc.com/news/uk-england–61227709, accessed 21 June 2022.

'everyday' or citizen heroes. The other two categories are slightly more complex. Seeger and Sellnow's analysis focuses on crises where first responders are deployed, such as in a natural or industrial disasters. The invasion in 1945 was a different type of crisis and so stories centre on the Germany army as rescuers in the crisis, rather than traditional first responders such as the fire service or police. The leader heroes are also less prominent as the leadership of the regime was either deemed criminal and/or blamed for the crisis. Despite these differences in characterisation hero narratives have similar function across crises as a source of comfort and hope. During Covid-19 the first responder model put forward by Seeger and Sellnow is represented in the heroization of medical staff. Among the everyday heroes in UK narratives an interesting character emerged – the 99-year-old WWII veteran fundraiser Captain Tom.[31] It is important to note that this chapter is not directly comparing the *Wehrmacht* to Captain Tom but rather highlights how stories of heroization circulate and their meaning for different societies in difficult times. In the Covid–19 pandemic leader heroes were easier to recognise and the leader of New Zealand Jacinda Arden was championed for her calm but decisive response to the crisis. Although these narratives are positive at first glance a more critical reading complicates their meaning demonstrating that it is important to look beyond initial representations of heroes and to think critically about the narratives.

Expellees tend to portray mothers and women as 'everyday heroes' and they are venerated for the adversity and violence endured during the 'crisis years' of 1943–48. Men were often absent due to the war, therefore, much of the struggles of daily life fell onto German women. Mothers are portrayed as being resourceful heroines for leading their family from danger and for their determination in ensuring their survival. One interviewee proudly recalled all of the troubles her mother had endured to ensure that her children first escaped the Soviet invasion and then to flee Communist East Germany.[32] Research into this topic has demonstrated that as a result of its association with Nazism, German masculinity was deemed problematic in the immediate post-war period.[33] Therefore, women became the symbols of the mid-to late 1940s and were portrayed as tirelessly striving to keep their families alive and as working to rebuild Germany from the ruins.[34] This is reflected in the

---

31 In the UK a range of groups fell into the everyday heroes category included key workers such as supermarket staff and lorry drivers.

32 Mr Kowald (German expellee), interviewed by Arddun Hedydd Arwyn, Neuenkirchen, Bremen, Germany, 5 November 2010, 01:08:00.

33 Robert G. Moeller, 'The "Remasculinization" of Germany in the 1950s: Introduction,' *Signs* 24, (1998): 101–6, 102.

34 Elizabeth Heineman, 'The Hour of the Woman: Memories of Germany's "Crisis Years" and West German National Identity,' *The American Historical Review*, 101:2 (1996), 354–395. Recently Leonie

narratives shared by displaced Germans and they demonstrate the need for heroes to provide comfort in the face of traumatic events.[35] The mother as a figure of a strength and individual resourcefulness is a powerful symbol of this need.[36]

German soldiers are also heroised in the narratives. They are portrayed as vanquished heroes who helped the refugees. Numerous accounts portray the kindness of soldiers supporting the image of the *Wehrmacht* as rescuers. These acts ranged from giving refugees lifts with military vehicles[37] to providing food and shelter.[38] Manfred Thomzik's narrative conveyed the impression that the *Wehrmacht* provided for – and protected – civilians as a part of their intrinsic duty. He wrote: 'All were thankful for this generosity, that they [the *Wehrmacht*] considered to be their duty.'[39] Recent research has demonstrated that the army had in fact made very little provision for the protection of civilians during the invasion as the military defence of East Prussia was their main priority. Civilians therefore directly suffered due to the army's actions.[40] Nevertheless, they have been mythologised as heroes in the stories shared about them.

There are also portrayals of the army as a heroic but defeated force. Heinz Buchholz, a young boy at the time, in particular offered numerous accounts of the brave *Wehrmacht* who had been let down by the treacherous Nazi party.[41] He commended their bravery as the 'unknown heroes' who had fought to provide

---

Treber has complicated the view of the heroized 'Rubble Women/Trummerfrauen' of postwar Germany by providing an integrated discussion of their backgrounds and work across the Zones of occupation: Leonie Treber, *Mythos Trümmerfrauen : von der Trümmerbeseitigung in der Kriegs – und Nachkriegszeit und der Entstehung eines deutschen Erinnerungsortes* (Essen: Klartext, 2015).

35 See also Seeger & Sellnow, *Narratives*, 113.

36 However, yet again this representation is more complex than initially thought. Recent work has problematized the role of women as saviors demonstrating that many were involved in crimes of the regime. See Leonie Treber, *Mythos Trümmerfrauen : von der Trümmerbeseitigung in der Kriegs – und Nachkriegszeit und der Entstehung eines deutschen Erinnerungsortes* (Essen: Klartext, 2015).

37 Greta Suck-Uring interviewed by Arddun Arwyn, Frau Suck-Uring, interviewed by AHA, 26 November, 2010 01:28:58; Manfred Thomzik, *Nur Der Gewinner Hat Recht : Wie Ein Ostpreuße Im Westen Ankommt*, 1. Aufl (Berlin: Frieling, 2009), 14.

38 Thomzik, *Nur der Gewinner hat Recht*, 20 and 46; Gregor Bergmann, *Mit Kopf Und Herz : Mein Weiter Weg Ins Leben* (Self–published, 2006), 75 & 95; Also: Irmgart Williams, interviewed by Arddun Arwyn, 19 January 2010, 00:05:38.

39 Thomzik, *Nur der Gewinner hat Recht*, 20.

40 Helmuth Greiner and Percy Ernst Schramm, *Kriegstagebuch Des Oberkommandos Der Wehrmacht (Wehrmachtführungsstab), 1940–1945*, vol. IV (München: Bernard & Graefe, 1982), 1325; Bastiaan Willems, *Violence in Defeat: The Wehrmacht on German Soil, 1944–1945* (Cambridge, United Kingdom ; New York, NY: Cambridge University Press, 2021), 207.

41 Heinz Buchholz, *Iwan, Das Panjepferd : Eine Kindheit Zwischen Krieg Und Frieden* (Hamburg: WWA-Verlag, 2002), 84–85.

refugees with an extra few hours to escape the 'advancing Russian-steamroller'[42] This portrayal embodies post-war myths about the German army that painted them as 'untainted' and 'honourable', distinct from the criminal Nazi regime and as innocent of genocide. Conversely the SS were held solely responsible for the crimes of the regime. These widely held myths were challenged by historians working in the 1990s and 2000s who conclusively demonstrated that the army took part directly in war crimes.[43] Accounts by expellees reflect the myths about the 'untainted' Wehrmacht and despite the narratives stemming from a period when those myths were being dispelled individuals rarely reflect badly on the army.[44] This demonstrates how narratives are important in creating and maintaining myths even in the face of overwhelming evidence to the contrary. It also draws attention to the pervasiveness of hero narratives and the role they play in giving meaning and providing hope during a crisis.

Hero narratives were also an important source of hope during the Covid-19 crisis. Medical staff became the centre of such narratives globally, with doctors, nurses and support staff not only working tirelessly but also contracting the virus and dying. In the UK the NHS was thanked in a multitude of ways. Landmarks were lit blue, businesses offered discounts to NHS staff, countrywide homes and streets were adorned with messages of support and the rainbow became the symbol of gratitude. Emulating countries that had gone into lockdown earlier Brits took to ritual clapping on a Thursday evening to express gratitude and feel solidary. The heroes in both sets of narratives became the protectors of the nation and representations of hope and survival - despite the great differences in their circumstances and actions. In both cases it is important to treat narratives critically and to look for what is being obscured. The heroization of the NHS obscured the failures of government and created a sense of inevitability in the way the pandemic was unfolding. Politicians supported the various acts heroizing the NHS as it drew attention away from their failures, such as delaying introducing a lockdown and the shortages of protective equipment.[45] The work undertaken by the

---

42 Heinz Buchholz, *Iwan, Das Panjepferd*, 109.

43 Detlev Bald, Johannes Klotz, and Wolfram Wette, *Mythos Wehrmacht. Nachkriegsdebatten und Traditionspflege.*, 1st edition (Berlin: Aufbau Taschenbuch, 2001); Hannes Heer et al., *The Discursive Construction of History. Remembering the Wehrmacht's War of Annihilation* (Basingstoke: Palgrave Macmillan, 2008).

44 Very few accounts are critical of German soldiers and are mostly sympathetic and grateful to them. A rare interview that does discuss German soldiers stealing was with Laura Martin and Renate Tepel, interviewed by Arddun Arwyn, 14 July 2010, 00:16:58.

45 Jennifer Mathers and Veronica Kitchen, 'NHS "Heroes" Should Not Have To Risk Their Lives To Treat Coronavirus Patients,' *The Conversation*, 20 April 2020, https://theconversation.com/nhs-her oes-should-not-have-to-risk-their-lives-to-treat-coronavirus-patients-136443, accessed 22 June 2022.

medical services during the pandemic was indeed heroic and their celebration was an important point of unity during dark times. However, we must always question whilst celebrating and seek deeper understandings beyond the overt hero narrative if we are to hold authorities accountable.

An everyday hero to emerge during the first months of lockdown was Captain Tom Moore, an elderly man whose charity walk for the NHS catapulted him into international stardom. Again, this example of a hero narrative provides comfort from knowing that 'everyday' people can achieve the extraordinary. Captain Tom had planned to raise £5,000 for an NHS charity by walking 100 lengths of his garden. When the press picked up on his attempts the story spread fast globally. Things did not end there. By the time the fund raiser had ended over £30 million was donated, and he was hailed as uniting the nation in times of darkness.[46] The honours and successes kept rolling in with a number one chart song, bestselling autobiography, knighthood, numerous awards and accolades, an honorary doctorate, murals, a bronze statue being awarded and dedicated to him. He even received a fly by from the Royal Airforce.[47]

If we consider the narratives constructed around Captain Tom (as opposed to the acts he undertook) we can also deconstruct some of the meanings that shape those stories and uncover what they tell us about how Britain sees itself in the early twenty-first century. Hero narratives are considered by scholars to be as much a reflection of the culture and beliefs of the society that venerates them, as they are about the hero themselves.[48] In a country, obsessed with the Second World War Captain Tom cut the perfect hero. Public memory of the war paints Britain as an underdog nation which prevailed through a stoic and plucky resilience, turning defeats into victories. In a time of crisis existing narratives about British resilience could be projected onto Captain Tom, a veteran and underdog due to his seniority who nevertheless valiantly battled against the odds to

---

46 The Captain Tom Foundation's website uses the term 'an ordinary man' to describe him. 'A World Without Ageism,' *The Captain Tom Foundation*, https://captaintom.org, accessed 9 August 2022.

47 Helen Burchell, 'Capt. Sir Tom Moore: How the Retired Army Officer Became A Nation's Hero,' *BBC News*, 2 February 2021, https://www.bbc.com/news/uk-england-beds-bucks-herts-52324058, accessed 9 August 2022; Anon., 'Captain Tom Becomes Cranfield University Honorary Graduate', Cranfield University, https://www.cranfield.ac.uk/press/news-2020/captain-tom-becomes-cranfield-university-honorary-graduate, accessed 9 August 2022; Anon., 'Captain Sir Tom Moore Bronze Statue Goes On Display For First Time In Leeds Retail Park,' *ITV News*, 1 May 2021, https://www.itv.com/news/calendar/2021-04-30/care-homes-across-spalding-honour-captain-toms-birthday-fund raiser, accessed 9 August 2022.

48 Max Jones, 'What Should Historians Do With Heroes? Reflections on Nineteenth – and Twentieth–Century Britain,' *History Compass* 5:2 (2007): 439–40.

prevail.[49] The raising of Captain Tom as a national hero of course stands in stark contrast to the way in which other elderly people were being treated in care homes. On one hand seniors were role models as the valiant heroes of war whilst at the same time bad government policies directly led to their deaths. Again, here we must be critical of what is being obscured by our veneration.

Finally, in the Covid-19 crisis the Prime Minister of New Zealand Jacinda Ardern emerged as a leader hero. In first half year of the crisis Jacinda Ardern received praise globally for her decisive containment of the virus in New Zealand through strict border controls and lockdowns. The hero narrative played out as the tale of a young, empathetic and sensible female leader that was able to safeguard her country. She was applauded for her direct, honest and empathetic communication during the crisis, where she both appeared unflappable but also sympathetic to the suffering of the nation.[50] This often stood in stark contrast to narratives of other countries that, led by bombastic and incompetent men, were being ravaged by the virus. To many, particularly on the political left, Jacinda and her success in containing the virus became a beacon of competence.[51] Seeger and Sellnow cite taking decisive action to reduce harm as central to the leader hero narrative. The display of calm, resoluteness and stability are also key tenets of the hero narrative.[52] In the Covid-19 crisis the hero leader narrative worked in conjunction with blame narratives. The figure of competent leadership is held up in direct opposition to perceived incompetence and poor decision making.

---

49 Not all stories end well, and the foundation set up in Tom's name has since come under scrutiny for some of its administrative and managerial practices. See: Anon., "UK Watchdog Investigates Captain Tom Charity," *Reuters*, 30 June 2022, https://www.reuters.com/world/uk/uk-watchdog-investigates-captain-tom-charity-2022-06-30/, accessed 9 August 2022; Anon., "Captain Tom 'charity' Autobiography Publisher Refuses To Say If Funds Paid To His Foundation From Sales," *The Independent*, 15 July 2022, https://www.independent.co.uk/news/uk/captain-tom-book-charity-b2123203.html, accessed 9 August 2022.

50 Uri Friedman, 'New Zealand's Prime Minister May Be the Most Effective Leader on the Planet,' *The Atlantic,* 19 April 2020, https://www.theatlantic.com/politics/archive/2020/04/jacinda-ardern-new-zealand-leadership-coronavirus/610237/, accessed on 23 June 2022.

51 Michaela J. Kerrissey and Amy C. Edmondson, 'What Good Leadership Looks Like During This Pandemic,' *Harvard Business Review,* 13 April 2020, https://hbr.org/2020/04/what-good-leadership-looks-like-during-this-pandemic, accessed on June 23, 2022. Ardern has received some criticism with regards to Covid policy and its impact of people of colour in New Zealand: Morgan Godfery, 'By Ending Covid Elimination, Jacinda Ardern Once Again Fails To Turn Compassion Into Policy,' *The Guardian*, 4 October 2021, https://www.theguardian.com/world/commentisfree/2021/oct/05/by-ending-covid-elimination-jacinda-ardern-once-again-fails-to-turn-compassion-into-policy, accessed on 23 June 2022.

52 Seeger & Sellnow, *Narratives*, 102.

Hero, victim and blame narratives of crisis are often closely related and inter-twined. They highlight positive and negative responses and actions, as evidenced in the case of the expellees and Covid-19. The function of hero narratives is to provide hope and comfort by offering models of good behaviour, valour and self-sacrifice for a greater good. This is important in creating unity and encouraging others to emulate such behaviour. One of the most important lessons that can be learned is to treat hero narratives critically and to search for what is being ob-scured by our focus on good deeds. In both cases there were examples of the hero narrative drawing attention away from darker realities.

Renewal Narratives

These types of narratives focus on rebuilding, improvement, and regeneration in the wake of a crisis[53] and they provide a narrative of a 'fresh start' following a di-sastrous event.[54] Expellees played an important role in the narratives of renewal in West Germany in the 1950s, and thereafter, due to their successful economic inte-gration into West German society. Despite their successful economic integration their social integration took much longer – if indeed it occurred at all. This case highlights the competing nature of narratives of crisis and renewal by demonstrat-ing how 'official' government narratives differ from individual experience.[55] In terms of the UK's recovery from the Covid-19 pandemic we can also recognise a divergence between government narratives of renewal and individual experience.

The year 1945 has often been simplistically portrayed as a breaking point with the past in Germany when Nazism and its causes was expunged from society. However, this idea has been questioned by scholars who argue that the continuity and changes before and after the end of the war were more complex than a simple break with the past.[56] Practically, it was impossible for a whole society to just change overnight and for everyone guilty of involvement with Nazism to dissolve

---

53 Timothy L. Sellnow and Matthew Seeger, *Narratives of Crisis: Telling Stories of Ruin and Re-newal* (Stanford: Stanford University Press, 2016), 81.

54 Brooke Fisher Liu et al., 'Telling the Tale: The Role of Narratives in Helping People Respond to Crises,' *Journal of Applied Communication Research* 48, no. 3 (2020): 330, https://doi.org/10.1080/00909882.2020.1756377.

55 Seeger and Sellow demonstrate competing narratives are a common element of narratives of crisis and that over time a process of convergence of narratives occurs. Seeger & Sellnow, *Narratives*, 81.

56 See Geoffrey J Giles, ed., *Stunde Null: The End and the Beginning Fifty Years Ago* (Washington, D.C.: German Historical Institute, 1997).

into thin air.[57] As the need to rebuild took precedent over all else, numerous former Nazis were given important roles in West German society and politics.[58] Yet despite these continuities a strong narrative of renewal was conjured in West Germany.[59] As a result of the huge economic successes of the 1950s this narrative became the West German 'economic miracle'. Through hard work and a focus on the future West Germany had risen from the ashes to become an economic powerhouse and reliable Cold War ally to the West.[60]

Expellee narratives fit neatly into the story of the economic miracle and have become an important part of the founding myth of West Germany. Expellees had lost everything yet through hard work, perseverance, and the support of the government, they were able to integrate economically. By looking at the themes discussed in autobiographical accounts economic integration can be considered an important marker in their journey. Most suffered from great economic hardships in the post-war era with many living in temporary accommodation for years. Often their post-war experience is the beginning of a narrative of renewal where they progress from dire poverty to economic stability usually through education and hard work.

Christa Wels, a young East Prussian woman, was housed in a refugee camp in West Germany after her expulsion from East Prussia. Such was her desperation to leave the camp she married a man she was fond of but did not love to get an apartment. Throughout the rest of her narrative, she discusses her self-improvement through learning to sew and eventually became a manager of a big garment firm. She struggled in her life with the traumas she underwent as a refugee but was able

---

57 Denazification was a notoriously difficult if not impossible task, see: Frederick Taylor, *Exorcising Hitler: The Occupation and Denazification of Germany* (New York: Bloomsbury Press, 2011).
58 See Norbert Frei, *Adenauer's Germany and the Nazi Past: The Politics of Amnesty and Integration, Adenauer's Germany and the Nazi Past* (New York ; Chichester: Columbia University Press, 2002), https://doi.org/10.7312/frei11882. The case of Hans Globke is covered by a Sunday Times podcast and article. Globke was an important figure in post-1949 West German government but had also been instrumental in the development of the anti-Sematic Nuremburg Laws: Oliver Moody, "Hans Globke, Hitler's Former Henchman, Was True Architect Of Modern Germany," *The Sunday Times*, 4 March 2021, https://www.thetimes.co.uk/article/hans-globke-hitlers-former-henchman-was-true-architect-of-modern-germany-7sw76fvkd, accessed on 11 August 2022.
59 Robert G. Moeller, 'The Politics of the Past in the 1950s: Rheotrics of Victimisation in East and West Germany,' in *Germans as Victims: Remembering the Past in Contemporary Germany*, ed. William John Niven (Basingstoke, Hampshire: Palgrave Macmillan, 2006), 35.
60 Elizabeth Heineman, 'The Hour of the Women: Memories of "Germany's Crisis" Year and West German National Identity,' in *The Miracle Years: A Cultural History of West Germany, 1949–1968*, ed. Hanna Schissler (Princeton: Princeton University Press, 2001), 35.

to gain some stability and fulfilment through economic success.[61] These kinds of journeys from destitute to stable homeowner with a successful career are common in the refugee narratives. They reflect individual experiences but are also coloured by the post-war West German economic success story of rebuilding and renewal.

Nevertheless, narratives of successful economic integration obscure deeper feelings of dislocation and homesickness.[62] Many found themselves in an ambiguous space where they understood that they could never return but also longed for an idealized place and time that no longer existed, and indeed had never existed.[63] Some experienced social discrimination all the way into the 1960s. For example, when Greta Suck-Uhring, who had fled East Prussia as a young child in 1945, wanted to marry a 'native' (German from West Germany) she faced anti-expellee prejudice from his family. This occurred in the 1960s demonstrating the longevity of bigotry held against expellees.[64] Others feel betrayed, as they feel they have disproportionally paid for the wider crimes of Germany. Manfred Neumann, who fled East Prussia in 1945, felt the Germans expellees suffered the greatest losses as a result of the war compared to other Germans. He stated '[those] who were here in the West, what did they even lose?'[65] There are numerous other examples of this bitterness that starkly contradicts the narratives of successful renewal through economic integration, demonstrating that narratives of renewal are more complex than face value. Something which is also evident in the Covid-19 narratives.

Narratives of renewal have already began to shape our understanding of the Covid-19 pandemic. 'Build, Back, Better' was the slogan adopted by British Prime Minister Boris Johnson to describe the government's Covid-10 recovery plan. The government narrative of renewal sought to improve and 'level up' British society. In a November 2021 speech Johnson called for addressing inequality in society and to prepare for the next looming crisis of climate change.[66] Under the 'Build, Back Better' slogan Johnson used the Victorian past to paint Britain as a country of science, technology and entrepreneurship. Drawing on the successful implementation of the Covid-19 vaccination in the UK Johnson wove a narrative of Britain's historic

---

61 Christel Wels like many other expellees went through multiple displacements. Having been stuck in East Prussia until 1948 living under Soviet rule she was deported to the German Democratic Republic from where she fled from to the Federal Republic in 1953. Christel Wels, *Der Unvergessene Weg : Eine Ostpreußische Biografie* (Berlin: Frieling, 2007), 85–108.

62 Kossert, *Kalte Heimat*, 13–14.

63 Andrew Demshuk, *The Lost German East : Forced Migration and the Politics of Memory, 1945–1970* (New York: Cambridge University Press, 2012), 13.

64 Greta Suck-Uring, interviewd by Arddun Arwyn, 26 November 2010, 02:14:15.

65 Manfred Neumann, interviewed by Arddun Arwyn, 2 October 2010, 01:52:24.

66 "G7: Boris Johnson kicks off summit with plea to tackle inequality," BBC News, 11 June 2021, https://www.bbc.com/news/uk-politics-57445184, accessed 23 June 2022.

place as a world leader in industry and development.[67] By the spring of 2022 the longer-term effects of the Covid-19 pandemic, such as inflation and slower economic growth, compounded with the Russian invasion of Ukraine and soaring energy prices resulting in serious global economic uncertainty, which compounded with the fallout of Brexit and severely impacted British households.[68] The most vulnerable, of course, have borne the brunt of the raise in living costs. In the narratives of everyday people struggling to warm their homes and feed their children, little comfort is drawn from grandiose references to a greater past. Instead, renewal is barely felt as years of austerity, the pandemic, Brexit and a global economic and environmental crisis bite. At the time of writing in early summer 2022 broader narratives of renewal are yet to develop and so we shall have to wait and see what the longer-term emotional impacts of the pandemic are beyond the initial grief of loss and effects of isolation.

The central lesson here is to be critical of narratives of renewal as they often reflect the needs of the government and organisations. By viewing crisis and overcoming through multiple lenses, such as the wider emotional needs of a community as well as economic renewal, we can look beyond and be critical of 'top-down' narratives. We are also able to build better understandings of how societies rebuild after crisis and that the emotional recovery from crises can take much longer and that they need to be addressed differently to economic recovery.

Memorial Narratives

Seeger and Sellnow's final strand of narratives of crisis are memorial narratives. These narratives have a public function and help societies draw longer term meanings.[69] Memorial narratives are also usually contested and competitive, and their meanings shift over time, but are ultimately about healing.[70] We can also

---

67 UK Government, Her Majesty's Treasury, *Build, Back Better: Our Plan for Growth*, 3 March 2021, https://www.gov.uk/government/publications/build-back-better-our-plan-for-growth/build-back-better-our-plan-for-growth-html, accessed on 23 June 2022. However, he failed to mention the well-documented social and economic inequalities of Victorian Britain and the role of his own party in perpetuating inequalities post-2008 through their austerity programme.

68 Larry Elliot, 'UK Economic Recovery At Risk From Rising Inflation And Waning Business Confidence,' *The Guardian*, 24 March 2022, https://www.theguardian.com/business/2022/mar/24/uk-economic-recovery-at-risk-from-rising-inflation-and-waning-business-confidence, accessed on 24 June 2022.

69 Liu et al., "Telling the Tale," 330.

70 Seeger & Sellnow, *Narratives of Crisis*, 129.

recognise such features in the memorial narratives of displacement from Eastern Europe. Changes to how victimhood is remembered has resulted in the development of divergent narratives about the past in Germany. The unfolding memorial narratives of the Covid-19 pandemic commemorate different types of victims and heroes and provide space for renewal. Despite these narratives being relatively young they have also been subject to contention.

Memorial narratives have been central to the discourse surrounding expellees. In the 1950s the memory of the expulsions played a role in public discourse about the war. This impetus came both from the West German government and the expellee organisations. The memorial narrative of the expulsions was represented in diverse spaces, from memorials to postage stamps and even street names. Small 'Heimat' or 'homeland' museums that commemorated the regions from which they had been expelled were also developed in West German town and cities.[71] Such museums provide a particularly fruitful area of study for understanding how memorial narratives are contested and change over time. Museums initially run by amateurs have been taken over by professional and state sponsored museums resulting in shifts in the narratives portrayed by exhibitions.[72]

Interestingly, these museums focussed less on the memory of fleeing in the narratives they conveyed and were instead more engaged with the memory of home before 1945. Most of the amateur run museums displayed disparate objects from the East and portrayed a narrative of home that uncritically reflected local cultures, economy and life. Objects range from those representing everyday life, such as family bibles, school graduation programmes and farm machinery, to representations of culture often portrayed through local costumes and regional peculiarities. The memorial narrative the museums portray is one-dimensional representation of life before 1945 which completely obscures difficult socio-economic and political realities. The biggest charge against them is their failure to represent crimes of the Third

---

71 Small regional museums like these have existed in Germany since the nineteenth century and have traditionally been a means of celebrating distinct local cultures. The practice was continued by expelled Germans from the former East who set up museums (of varying size and quality) across West Germany commemorating the regions and towns from which they had been expelled. See Cornelia Eisler, '"State-Supported History" at the Local Level: Ostdeutsche Heimatstuben and Expellee Museums in West Germany,' in *The Palgrave Handbook of State-Sponsored History After 1945*, ed. Berber Bevernage and Nico Wouters (London: Palgrave Macmillan UK, 2018), 399–413, https://doi.org/10.1057/978-1-349-95306-6_21; Andrew Demshuk, 'Godfather Cities: West German Patenschaften and the Lost German East*,' *German History* 32, no. 2 (June 1, 2014): 224–55.

72 Arddun Hedydd Arwyn, '"Cystadlaethau Cof", Naratif a Hanes Yn Amgueddfa "Heimat" Wehlau: Negodi Hanes a Chof Cymhleth Yr Almaen Yn Yr Ugeinfed Ganrif," *Gwerddon*, 2017, 68–69, https://pure.aber.ac.uk/portal/files/39656228/Gwerddon25_e3.pdf.

Reich, the Holocaust and the war. The flight and expulsions are sometimes represented, usually through luggage, but there is often no explanation of how these events occurred (reflecting the earlier narratives of blame and victimhood).

Memorial narratives are both contested and change over time,[73] and this is also the case with the narratives portrayed in the museums. In the 1960s the narratives of victimhood surrounding the expulsions began to be challenged, which led to the memorial narratives of the 1950s being questioned by West Germans, particularly by the younger generation who were born after Nazism. Increasingly, the Holocaust became the principal memory of the war, resulting in the singular memory of German victimhood, often associated with the expulsions, becoming less dominant. In line with these changes to the broader memory culture, the Heimat museums with their nostalgic and one-sided representations became out of date. As the world changed around them the Heimat museums remain(ed) largely static and out of touch with broader West German society. As time has progressed and the custodians of these museums slowly pass away, they are closed or are subsumed by larger museums. This results in the reinterpretation of the narratives within them to reflect contemporary understandings of the past. These are more critical and portray the more complex elements of Germany's history, including German complicity in the Holocaust.[74] Memorial narratives of crisis are often those which have the longest legacy as they come to represent the meaning of the crisis in the long term. In the case of the narratives of displacement they have become contested over time with divergent narratives developing between those who experienced the flight and the mainstream of German society.

Even in the first year of the pandemic memorial narratives began to emerge which reflect some of the tropes discussed above. A bronze memorial depicting stoic health and key workers and a hunched elderly man opened in November 2021 in Barnsley. The statue draws on the 'hero health worker' narrative and on the victimhood of the elderly.[75] The relationship between different types of narratives (hero and victim) are evident in this example. A wooden temple built in Bedworth, Warwickshire displays both a memorial and renewal narrative. The sculpture of an ornate temple was designed to be burnt shortly after its completion. The opportunity to add messages of commemoration to the sculpture was given to the public before it was set ablaze in May 2021. Designers emphasised the cathartic nature of

---

73 Sellnow and Seeger, *Narratives of Crisis*, 128.

74 Arwyn, "'Cystadlaethau Cof,'" 59–60.

75 Anon., 'Covid Memorial Sculpture Unveiled In Barnsley,' BBC News, 22 November 2021, https://www.bbc.com/news/uk-england-south-yorkshire-59373781, accessed 24 June 2022.

the endeavour with the ritualised burning symbolising letting go and creating space for renewal.[76]

In spring 2021 an unofficial national memorial sprang up directly opposite the Houses of Parliament that sought to commemorate the victims of the pandemic through individually painted hearts. This memorial represented the victim narrative and focussed on individuality whilst concurrently representing the scale of deaths.[77] The memorial also had a political message and was created *by Covid-19 Bereaved Families for Justice*, a group calling for governmental accountability and for an official enquiry into the government's handling of the pandemic. Therefore, behind the memorial narrative we can also recognise blame narratives. The UK government is yet to designate a national day and space for remembrance but it will be interesting to see, when the time comes, how it will approach the commemoration and how it will attempt to reconcile competing narratives of heroism, victimhood and blame. Whatever the outcome, it will no doubt reflect a narrative favourable to the government in power at that time.

As can be deduced from both examples, memorial narratives shape the commemoration of a crisis and they provide spaces for reflection, remembrance and comfort. They are however, also often shaped by the needs of a particular group, be it political or simply cathartic. It is important that we, therefore, stop and question the types of representation in memorial narratives to seek out and understand its function. A further interesting lesson is that memorial narratives change over time. As can be seen from the example of the German expellees. The memorial narratives of the crisis are very much shaped by the culture and values of the present. Therefore, the Covid memorial narratives are currently shaped by the ongoing calls for accountability as well as the grief of those who have lost loved ones. Over time the way in which the pandemic is remembered will be shaped by perceptions at the time it is being memorialised. We can only hope that the memorial narratives help shape future crisis management and disaster preparedness as well as ensuring that similar failures are avoided in the future.

---

76 Anon., 'Burning Date For Covid Memorial In Bedworth Announced', BBC News, 18 May 2022, https://www.bbc.com/news/uk-england-coventry-warwickshire-61482163, accessed 24 June 2022.

77 Kevin Rawlinson, 'Covid Bereaved Begin Work On Memorial Wall Opposite Westminster,' *The Guardian*, 29 March 2021, https://www.theguardian.com/world/2021/mar/29/covid-bereaved-begin-work-memorial-wall-opposite-westminster, accessed 24 June 2022; Pan Pylas, 'Art Therapy: How UK's COVID Memorial Wall Brought Comfort,' *Associated Press News*, 30 October 2021, https://apnews.com/article/coronavirus-pandemic-europe-health-pandemics-london-bfddccafdcb9a3135a75b5cb65751da3, accessed 24 June 2022.

Conclusions

It is striking that it has been possible to identify each of the tropes outlined by Seeger and Sellnow in the narratives of both cases, despite their very different nature. This suggests that patterns exist in the ways that we as humans tell stories about crises and that these narratives can provide clear lessons. First and foremost, a resounding lesson to be learned is that we need to be critical of narratives in all their forms. By teaching individuals to search for tropes in the narratives they consume, they can begin to make informed reactions to information and think critically about how a crisis is being depicted. In this age of social media emotional reactions to news and information has been exploited by algorithms purposely seeking to induce emotional responses contributing to misinformation spreading quickly. As a means of combating base responses understanding patterns and archetypes in stories can help the individual place a distance between the story and their response. For example, if individuals better understood how blame narratives operate, they may respond less emotionally to narratives that stigmatise certain groups and instead can learn evaluate the information critically.

It is also clear that narratives are a significant source of comfort in times of crisis. Hero, renewal and memorial narratives are important in providing meaning in situations which often seem out of one's control. It is evident that individuals reach for existing and shared patterns of narration when undergoing crisis to provide comfort and reassurance, hope and optimism. Such narratives also need to be considered critically as there are often more complicated realities behind the narrative. These narratives can also be used to provide insights into the society that propagates them. By analysing the content of the narratives, we can find clues about the society and the time in which the narratives are shared.

The final lesson is that narratives are important in creating unity among a group. Each of Seeger and Sellnow's themes has brought people together through their shared understanding of the crisis expressed through a narrative. We saw this in blame, victim and hero narratives where they often intersect and create a basis for group solidarity especially in the immediate aftermath. In the longer-term renewal and memorial narratives are also significant in creating group solidarity and were important, alongside the other narrative types, in calls for restitution and accountability.

Understanding narratives is central to the meanings that we take from crises and has significant impacts on how societies choose to allocate resources, both material and cultural, to overcoming crisis. The ways in which we talk about crises are crucial to the process of coming to terms, building new societies from the rubble and avoiding such mistakes in the future. Gaining a better appreciation of how people respond to crisis through the stories they tell helps prepare us for future crisis as we can begin to anticipate how societies and individuals may react. Although narratives largely tell us more about how people perceive events rather than the actual event itself they are nevertheless very powerful – arguably more powerful than reality. As larger looming crises, such as climate change and the threat of further global pandemics, bear down on us we can learn from how past peoples have perceived crisis.

References

Ahonen, Pertti. 'Domestic Constraints on West German Ostpolitik: The Role of the Expellee Organizations in the Adenauer Era.' *Central European History* 31:1–2 (1998): 31–63. https://doi.org/10.1017/S0008938900016034.

Arwyn, Arddun Hedydd. '"Cystadlaethau Cof", Naratif a Hanes Yn Amgueddfa "Heimat" Wehlau: Negodi Hanes a Chof Cymhleth Yr Almaen Yn Yr Ugeinfed Ganrif.' *Gwerddon*, 2017. https://pure.aber.ac.uk/portal/files/39656228/Gwerddon25_e3.pdf.

Bald, Detlev, Johannes Klotz, and Wolfram Wette. *Mythos Wehrmacht. Nachkriegsdebatten und Traditionspflege*. 1st edition. Berlin: Aufbau Taschenbuch, 2001.

Bergmann, Gregor. *Mit Kopf Und Herz: Mein Weiter Weg Ins Leben*. Self-published, 2006.

Buchholz, Heinz. *Iwan, Das Panjepferd: Eine Kindheit Zwischen Krieg Und Frieden*. Hamburg: WWA-Verlag, 2002.

Connor, Ian. *Refugees and Expellees in Post-War Germany*. Manchester: Manchester University Press, 2007.

Demshuk, Andrew. "Godfather Cities: West German Patenschaften and the Lost German East*." *German History* 32: 2 (2014): 224–55. https://doi.org/10.1093/gerhis/ghu033.

Demshuk, Andrew. *The Lost German East: Forced Migration and the Politics of Memory, 1945–1970*. New York: Cambridge University Press, 2012.

Douglas, R. M. *Orderly and Humane: The Expulsion of the Germans after the Second World War*. New Haven: Yale University Press, 2012.

Eisler, Cornelia. '"State-Supported History" at the Local Level: Ostdeutsche Heimatstuben and Expellee Museums in West Germany.' In *The Palgrave Handbook of State-Sponsored History After 1945*, edited by Berber Bevernage and Nico Wouters, 399–413. London: Palgrave Macmillan UK, 2018. https://doi.org/10.1057/978-1-349-95306-6_21.

Frei, Norbert. *Adenauer's Germany and the Nazi Past: The Politics of Amnesty and Integration. Adenauer's Germany and the Nazi Past*. New York; Chichester: Columbia University Press, 2002. https://doi.org/10.7312/frei11882.

Giles, Geoffrey J, ed. *Stunde Null: The End and the Beginning Fifty Years Ago*. Washington, D.C.: German Historical Institute, 1997.

Greiner, Helmuth, and Percy Ernst Schramm. *Kriegstagebuch Des Oberkommandos Der Wehrmacht (Wehrmachtführungsstab), 1940–1945*. Vol. IV. München: Bernard & Graefe, 1982.

Hahn, Eva, and Hans Henning Hahn. *Die Vertreibung im deutschen Erinnern. Legenden, Mythos, Geschichte*. Paderborn: Verlag Ferdinand Schöningh, 2010.

Heer, Hannes, Walter Manoschek, Alexander Pollak, and Ruth Wodak. *The Discursive Construction of History. Remembering the Wehrmacht's War of Annihilation*. Basingstoke: Palgrave Macmillan, 2008.

Heineman, Elizabeth. 'The Hour of the Women: Memories of "Germany's Crisis" Year and West German National Identity.' In *The Miracle Years: A Cultural History of West Germany, 1949–1968*, edited by Hanna Schissler. Princeton: Princeton University Press, 2001.

Kossert, Andreas. *Kalte Heimat: Die Geschichte der deutschen Vertriebenen nach 1945*. Munich: Pantheon Verlag, 2009.

Liu, Brooke Fisher, Lucinda Austin, Yen-I Lee, Yan Jin, and Seoyeon Kim. 'Telling the Tale: The Role of Narratives in Helping People Respond to Crises.' *Journal of Applied Communication Research* 48:3 (2020): 328–49. https://doi.org/10.1080/00909882.2020.1756377.

Martin, Laura, and Renate Tepel. interviewed by Arddun Arwyn, 14 July 2010.

Moeller, Robert G. 'Sinking Ships, the Lost Heimat and Broken Taboos: Günter Grass and the Politics of Memory in Contemporary Germany.' *Contemporary European History* 12:2 (2003): 147–81. https://doi.org/10.1017/S0960777303001139.

Moeller, Robert G. 'The Politics of the Past in the 1950s: Rhetorics of Victimisation in East and West Germany.' In *Germans as Victims: Remembering the Past in Contemporary Germany*, edited by William John Niven. Basingstoke, Hampshire: Palgrave Macmillan, 2006.

Sellnow, Timothy L., and Matthew Seeger. *Narratives of Crisis: Telling Stories of Ruin and Renewal*. Stanford: Stanford University Press, 2016.

Taylor, Frederick. *Exorcising Hitler: The Occupation and Denazification of Germany*. New York: Bloomsbury Press, 2011.

Thomzik, Manfred. *Nur Der Gewinner Hat Recht: Wie Ein Ostpreuße Im Westen Ankommt*. 1. Aufl. Berlin: Frieling, 2009.

Wels, Christel. *Der Unvergessene Weg: Eine Ostpreußische Biografie*. Berlin: Frieling, 2007.

Willems, Bastiaan. *Violence in Defeat: The Wehrmacht on German Soil, 1944–1945*. Cambridge, United Kingdom: New York, NY: Cambridge University Press, 2021.

Williams, Irmgart. interviewed by Arddun Arwyn, 19 January 2010.

List of Contributors

Dr Arddun H. Arwyn is a Lecturer in Modern History at Aberystwyth University, Wales, specialising in twentieth century German history. Her current research project *The Refugee Journey. Liminality and Narrative in East Prussian Memories 1944-today* is centred on the forced migration of East Prussian Germans from Eastern Europe after the Second World War. The book explores the autobiographical narratives of East Prussians to uncover the broader meanings of their refugee journeys.

Dr Elizabeth Benjamin is Assistant Professor (Research) in Memory Studies at Coventry University, UK, and specialises in the modern and contemporary French and Francophone context. Her particular interests are the ways in which we choose to remember people, events, and things, and how we create narratives of inclusion and exclusion around them. She is interested in cultural manifestations of memory, and particularly monuments, literature, and visual culture.

Dr Iro Filippaki is a Medical Humanities researcher, focusing on literary representations of physical and mental trauma. After completing her graduate studies at the University of Glasgow, and a postdoctoral research post at Johns Hopkins University, Iro has returned to Athens, Greece where she currently teaches Medical Humanities and other interdisciplinary courses at the American College of Greece. She is also an editor for De Gruyter's book series Computer Games and the Humanities. Her monograph published in 2021 was titled The Poetics of Post-Traumatic Stress Disorder in Postmodern Literature, and her current research focuses on representations of resilience and impatient bodies in literature.

Dr Josephine Hoegaerts is Professor of European Culture after 1800 at the University of Amsterdam. Her work focuses on histories of vocal health and propriety as well as different modes of political speech in the nineteenth century. She has recently published (2021) 'Voices that Matter? Methods for Historians Attending to the Voices of the Past' in *Historical Reflections/Réflexions Historiques.* The article explores and considers interdisciplinary approaches to the history of voices and presents innovative ways to 'listen anew' to familiar sources.

Dr Franziska E. Kohlt is a researcher in the history and communication of science, and comparative literature, and currently a Leverhulme Research Fellow at the University of Leeds. Her research investigates the interactions between narrative, metaphor and analogy in science communication, the formation of public understandings of science and behaviour change, especially in scientific discourse conducted in media, literature and visual culture.

Dr Kristopher Lovell is Assistant Professor in History at Coventry University. He is predominantly a specialist in the relationship between politics and the media in wartime Britain (1939-1945). His PhD 'Press, Politics and the People's War', conducted at Aberystwyth University, was part of a research project funded by the Leverhulme Trust: A Social and Cultural History of the British Press in the Second World War. He has previously published work on the relationship between the British popular press and the Common Wealth Party and has a forthcoming monograph based on his PhD.

Dr Alexandra Palli is currently a Scientific collaborator at the University Mental Health, Neurosciences and Precision Medicine Research Institute. Their PhD, undertaken at the National and Kapodistrian University of Athens, explored the implementation and evaluation of psychoeducation

https://doi.org/10.1515/9783110731002-010

intervention in groups of family members. Their publications include multiple collaborations exploring rehabilitation and recovery from schizophrenia.

Dr Darren R. Reid is Assistant Professor in History at Coventry University. He specialises in the history of race, culture and indigeneity across the Americas. He has worked extensively with Indigenous peoples across Brazil, collaborating with them to produce new oral histories and autobiographical material. His recent research includes examining the impact of Covid-19 upon indigenous South Americans and he has recently published a book on Native American Racism in the Age of Donald Trump: Historical and Contemporary Perspectives (Palgrave, 2020).

Dr Christopher Smith has been a Lecturer in History at Coventry University since 2017. He is the author of two books, *The Hidden History of Bletchley Park* (2015) and *The Last Cambridge Spy* (2019). He is currently co-writing a book on the myth and memory of Bletchley Park with Dr Thomas Knowles. Before his appointment at Coventry, he taught history at the University of Kent, Bournemouth University, the University of Worcester and Aberystwyth University.

Dr Sarah Turner is Assistant Professor of Cognitive Linguistics in the Research Centre for Arts, Memory and Communities at Coventry University. Her research focuses on the analysis of figurative language production to provide insights into physical, psychological and social experiences, with a current focus on the experience of grief and bereavement. She is particularly interested in how individuals use language in creative ways to help them to understand, conceptualise and communicate their experiences, and how an analysis of such language can be used to inform better care.

Index

https://doi.org/10.1515/9783110731002-011